In Clinical Practice

Taking a practical approach to clinical medicine, this series of smaller reference books is designed for the trainee physician, primary care physician, nurse practitioner and other general medical professionals to understand each topic covered. The coverage is comprehensive but concise and is designed to act as a primary reference tool for subjects across the field of medicine.

More information about this series at http://www.springer.com/series/13483

Sami Shousha

Breast Pathology in Clinical Practice

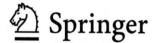 Springer

Sami Shousha (Deceased)
Imperial College
Imperial College Healthcare NHS Trust
London
UK

ISSN 2199-6652 ISSN 2199-6660 (electronic)
In Clinical Practice
ISBN 978-3-030-42385-8 ISBN 978-3-030-42386-5 (eBook)
https://doi.org/10.1007/978-3-030-42386-5

This Springer imprint is published by the registered company Springer Nature Switzerland AG
The registered company address is: Gewerbestrasse 11, 6330 Cham, Switzerland

*To Seham, Sarah, Susan
and Adam*

Memories of the Life and Achievements of Professor Shousha

These memories of Professor Sami Shousha have been collated by his wife, Seham Shousha, and his daughter, Sarah Shousha, to honour him. It is of deepest sadness to us all that Professor Shousha died from COVID-19 during the Coronavirus pandemic. Publication of this book meant a great deal to him and he had seen it through to final proof stages with his legendary dedication and enthusiasm. We are deeply grateful for his world-renowned expertise in the field of breast pathology and remember him also as a devoted family man and a truly beautiful human being who lived by the highest principles and values.

Professor Shousha lived his life with purpose; he was one of the most extraordinary doctors, scientists, academics, and pathologists of his generation. An exemplary consultant clinician and professor, his endless passion for his work and unrelenting professionalism were unsurpassed. He served the NHS with pride and dedication, showing considerable fortitude in the face of workplace pressures and staff shortages, and was a source of inspiration for many people. He worked until the last weeks of his life when he was nearly 80, long after others would have retired.

Professor Shousha graduated from Cairo University in 1964 and trained in histopathology at the Royal Free Hospital and the School of Medicine in London. In 1978 he joined Charing Cross Hospital, where he worked for the remainder of his career. He pursued his interest in breast disorders and specialised in the diagnosis and characterisation of these disorders. He was appointed an honorary Professor at Imperial College and served as the Clinical Lead for the breast histopathology service at Imperial College Healthcare NHS Trust.

Professor Shousha was a pioneering clinician, researcher, and educator as well as an expert in quality governance. His encyclopaedic knowledge of his field resulted in his reputation as an international expert on breast disorders. As his standing grew over the decades, he was always ready to go above and beyond and help the many acquaintances around the world who turned to him for advice; they remain forever grateful.

He wanted his patients to benefit from his in-depth knowledge of this microscopic disease; his commitment to them was absolute. Many thousands of people unknowingly benefited from his knowledge and the careful attention to detail that characterised his work. He took not just breast pathology to a new level, but all aspects of cellular pathology. His knowledge base and years of experience had a direct influence on standards of care.

Professor Shousha led many international symposia, delivered numerous stimulating keynote lectures, and took the lead role in piloting, researching, and standardising numerous laboratory tests in breast pathology. These include immunohistochemistry and in situ hybridisation. For well over a decade, he championed the pathology breast screening service at Charing Cross Hospital for the West of London, an NHS breast screening service that serves over 60,000 women. He provided an essential link between laboratory science and patients with breast cancer, co-authoring numerous publications in conjunction with the laboratory research team.

He undertook research in various aspects of diagnostic and prognostic breast parameters including receptors, tumour phenotype and behaviour, protein expression, and biology and treatment-related changes in a wide repertoire of breast tumours. Changes related to neo-adjuvant and triple-negative cancers were of particular interest to him. He dedicated a lot of time to working with scientists and PhD students to help develop a targeted treatment model. With over 300 scientific publications, ranging from peer-reviewed journal articles to book chapters and textbooks, his contribution to breast pathology and diagnostic and prognostic sciences was unrivalled.

His greatest joy, however, was in educating others. A gifted teacher, he relished in delivering sessions to all audiences, including medical students, biomedical scientists, consultants, and international visitors. He took great pleasure in hosting visiting scholars or fellows at Charing Cross. He would give everyone his undivided attention, no matter how junior or senior, and was always willing to share his vast archives, of which he was most proud. He taught with abundant humour and infectious enthusiasm; many trainee pathologists went on to specialise in breast pathology because of his influence.

Professor Shousha believed in people learning for themselves, rather than being taught. According to him, teaching was only one aspect of learning. His annual week-long Diagnostic Breast Pathology course at Charing Cross Hospital was always oversubscribed with fellow consultants from around the world and was highly valued. Sadly his death coincided with this year's course, something he had again worked so hard to organise. Also extremely popular were the annual conferences he ran in Egypt; year after year he tried, unsuccessfully, to step back from being a guest speaker. He was told however that his teaching was indispensable. Scores of medical and allied health care professionals, trainees, consultants, nurses, and students were privileged enough to be taught and trained by him over the decades.

Professor Shousha devoted much of his time to a number of worthy causes, including his role with the International Association of Pathology; he was the first in a long line of 'Visiting Goodwill Ambassadors' who provided education to the organisation's underserved divisions. He spent several days in the West Bank, giving lectures and seminars to medical students and graduates. He became a popular and highly esteemed speaker at The Arab Division of the Association, often invited to lecture at its annual scientific meeting. His family fondly remembers attending these, and other congresses, and being proud of his achievements and the ever-increasing number of lives he was so positively influencing.

Just a few weeks before he died, he showed oncologist colleagues around the new laboratories at Charing Cross Hospital; extensively equipped, these were his pride and joy and he had been key to their development. His death is a great loss for the pathology fraternity, the clinical and academic teams, and members of the breast pathology unit at Charing Cross. He leaves a large vacuum.

The Chief Executive of Imperial College Healthcare, Professor Tim Orchard, shares fond memories:

> 'We were so grateful for Sami's world-renowned expertise in the field of breast pathology. With his kind, caring nature, legendary dedication to work, and passion for teaching, he influenced the careers and touched the lives of so many people.'

It was, however, his modest and unassuming character that made him most special. His generous, gentle, and self-effacing personality was an example to us all. In the scores of cards, letters, and emails his family has recently received, many colleagues said they considered him an honourable, compassionate, and irreplaceable friend who looked out for others. His students said they considered him not just a mentor, but a father figure and supporter. He showed much love to those he tutored, some of whom had no family in the UK, offering them courage and strength on a personal and professional level.

A devoted husband, father, grandfather, friend, and colleague, he stood and lived by nothing but the highest of principles and values. Work was always highly important; right up to the end of his life, he would leave the house by 7 am and would often not return until after 8 pm. Nevertheless, Professor Shousha adored his family and liked nothing more than taking them on holiday and out for meals. There was of course the birth of his first grandchild, Adam, who looks just like him. May he follow in his footsteps, no pressure there! On the day of his grandchild's birth, he dropped his daughter at the hospital and then went to work. He only returned once he had completed his own essential engagements, but thankfully did make it back in time for the birth! His fondest recent memories include spending Adam's first birthday at Center Parcs and his own last birthday spent at a favourite family mansion house retreat. Seham, his wife, meant the world to him; one close friend says he admitted that she 'did everything' for him. He never had to worry about packing for a conference and felt much happier when she travelled with him. Indeed behind every great man…

Professor Shousha sacrificed a considerable amount of time during the last years of his life to this book. Draft versions went on many family holidays. He was unable to truly switch off as finishing this book to the highest standard meant a great deal to him. It often kept him awake at night. In fact, many of his final conversations when in hospital were about ensuring the publication of this book.

Professor Shousha is sorely missed and will always be treasured in our hearts. The world is a lesser place without him. May he be a role model to us all and may his goodness live on in us. May God have mercy on his soul and reward him for all he has done for humanity. His last words to his wife and daughter were that he did 'his best' in all aspects of his life. With these words we invite you, as readers, to share in his legacy and take it forward.

Contents

Introduction

The role of the Surgical Pathologist in dealing with breast diseases has changed enormously during the last few years. The introduction of mammographic screening, conservative breast surgery and core, vacuum-assisted and sentinel lymph node biopsies, have changed the type of material received by the Pathologist for diagnosis, and the type of information required from him. Requests for frozen sections have markedly diminished, but new challenges have arisen, particularly in respect of diagnosing border-line lesions which are being increasingly detected by mammography, confirming the complete excision of malignant lesions, interpreting core and vacuum-assisted biopsies and examining and reporting specimens from patients who had neo-adjuvant chemo or hormone therapy.

This book is based on my experience at Charing Cross Hospital, London; and is aimed at presenting concise practical information for practising and trainee pathologists. It can also be of interest to other clinical practitioners looking after patients with breast disease who would like to know how pathologists work to reach up a diagnosis on which management of the disease is based. It also provides those practitioners with a 'glossary' of terms used and names given to various breast lesions and what they mean. I have previously published some of the discussed aspects in several review articles [1–4] and in an edited book [5].

© Springer Nature Switzerland AG 2020   1
S. Shousha, *Breast Pathology in Clinical Practice*, In Clinical
Practice, https://doi.org/10.1007/978-3-030-42386-5_1

References

1. Shousha S. Histopathology of breast carcinoma and related conditions. In: Hoogstraten B, Burn I, Bloom HJG, editors. Breast cancer. Berlin: Springer; 1989. p. 13–44.
2. Shousha S. New aspects in the histological diagnosis of breast carcinoma. Semin Surg Oncol. 1996;12:12–25.
3. Shousha S. Reporting breast biopsies. Curr Diagn Pathol. 2000;6:140–5.
4. Shousha S. Issues in the interpretation of breast core biopsies. Int J Surg Pathol. 2003;11:167–76.
5. Shousha S, editor. Breast pathology. Problematic issues. Switzerland: Springer International Publishing; 2017.

Core Biopsy

The Patient

To be a good breast pathologist you have to put yourself in the position of the patient. She, as patients with breast disease are mostly women, is anxious and frightened; either because she herself has discovered a lump in her breast, or she was told, after a routine screening, that she has an abnormal area in her breast that needs further investigation. This entails introducing a needle in the breast to get a sample of the lesion for microscopic examination. The first thing that will come to the patent's mind would be the dreaded breast cancer. Whatever re-assuring the radiologist or surgeon is, the patient will not settle down until she is told the 'Pathologist's' confirmed diagnosis. Hence the need for a fast and accurate diagnosis.

The Lesion

This could be either a palpable mass or a non-palpable lesion in the breast that was discovered by radiology in the form of abnormal microcalcification, a shadow of a soft tissue mass or an area of architectural distortion. The patient might also have abnormal axillary lymph nodes that need examination. The abnormal lymph node may have been detected by palpation or by abnormal radiological appearance.

© Springer Nature Switzerland AG 2020

S. Shousha, *Breast Pathology in Clinical Practice*, In Clinical Practice, https://doi.org/10.1007/978-3-030-42386-5_2

The Doctor

Core biopsies are usually taken by Radiologists guided by x-ray, ultrasound, or less commonly, magnetic resonance imaging (MRI) machines. Surgeons sometimes do free, unaided, clinical cores for palpable lesions. Some Pathologists carry out fine needle aspirations.

The Needle

Hollow needles of different widths are used. Fine needles are used to get fluid aspirates from cysts or from patients who cannot tolerate the introduction of bigger needles. The most commonly used needle for getting a core biopsy, particularly for palpable lesions, is the 14 Gauge (G) needle. Needles with wider bores (11 or 10 G) are used with vacuum assistance, particularly for mammographic lesions with microcalcifications.

Type of Biopsies

Fine needle aspiration was the only technique available to get samples of breast lesions for microscopic examination until the introduction of core biopsies. It is mainly used now to aspirate cysts. The sample obtained usually contains some desquamated cells that can be examined microscopically to determine whether they are benign or malignant. The technique is also sometimes used to get samples from solid lesions in patients with bleeding disorders. Only a limited number of cells is obtained by this technique, and the amount of information provided can be very limited. Core biopsies are now the most widely used method for obtaining a non-operative/pre-operative diagnosis of breast lesions. They have superseded the use of fine needle aspiration cytology for that purpose mainly because of their higher specificity and sensitivity, their ability to differentiate, in most cases, between invasive and non-invasive, in situ, tumours, and because most pathologists are more familiar with diagnosing tissue sections, which a core can provide, than dealing with cytology preparations.

Stereotactic biopsies are taken by Radiologists using mammograms with a stereotactic attachment that can pinpoint the location of the radiologic abnormality, mostly microcalcifications, and accurately direct the core biopsy needle to it. Local anaesthetic is applied and a small incision is made in the skin before the introduction of the needle or the vacuum assisted probe.

Ultrasound guided core biopsies are also usually taken by Radiologists using an ultrasound device that produces accurate image of the structure of the breast. This helps accurate localisation of the abnormal area where the needle can then be inserted to get the required samples from the lesion. x-rays can be taken to show the needle within the lesion.

MRI guided biopsies are less commonly used usually to locate or exclude the presence of suspected lesions that were not seen using the other above-mentioned methods. MRI captures multiple cross sectional images of the breast and then combines them, using a computer, to generate a detailed three-diminsional images that can localise minute areas of abnormalities in the breast. The technique is so sensitive that not-uncommonly would pick up slightly worrying lesions that later prove to be benign by microscopic examination.

Either fine needle aspiration or an ultrasound guided core biopsy can be used for getting samples from abnormal lymph nodes.

The Sample

If the core biopsy was carried out for microcalcification, the radiologist should x-ray the cores to confirm the presence of calcification in them [1]. It would be useful if the cores' x-ray is available for the pathologist to review, either digitally or as a hard copy, or at least for the radiologist to mention in the request form that the presence of calcification in the cores has been confirmed. It may be also useful to provide the cores containing calcium in a sepa-

rate container, so that they can be embedded separately and if calcification is not seen microscopically in the first few sections,
further sections can be cut from this particular paraffin block. The
number of cores taken usually depends on the size and type of
lesion, whether it is a mass or an area of calcification, as well as
on the size of the needle used. It has been found that for stereotactic 14-gauge needle biopsy, 5 cores will achieve diagnosis of 99%
of masses and 6 cores will lead to a diagnosis in 92% of microcalcification cases [2]. More cores have to be taken if the x-ray shows
no microcalcification in the removed ones. A higher percentage of
diagnosis in microcalcification cases can be achieved by using the
11 or 10-gauge vacuum-assisted device [3]. The cores should be
dropped in formalin immediately after removal to ensure proper
fixation.

The Request Form

The biopsy should be sent to the Pathology Laboratory with a
completed request form carrying the patient's full information,
the reason for carrying the biopsy, the technique used, the number
of cores and the suspected diagnosis. It is also important to indicate in the form the degree of suspicion, in a scale varying from 1
to 5, where 1 is probably normal and 5 is highly suspicious of
malignancy. The prefix P is used if the degree of suspicion was
based on clinical examination, M if based on mammography and
U if based on ultrasound. Figure 2.1 shows an example of a
request form used in our institution.

The Laboratory

In the pathology Lab, for each case the number of cores received,
their length and colour is recorded. All cores are processed, preferably not more than four cores in each cassette. We cut three
shallow levels from each paraffin block for staining with haema-
toxlyn and eosin (H&E). We keep three intervening sections
unstained to be used for immunohistochemistry if needed. Usually

WEST OF LONDON BREAST SCREENING SERVICE
ASSESSMENT BIOPSY FORM

DATE PERFORMED:_____
Time of Biopsy:_____
Client's Gender: Female

RADIOLOGIST: _____

Surname:	
Name:	
DOB:	
ECX:	

Please affix assessment label here

MAMMOGRAM

Right

☐ Asymmetry
☐ Distortion
☐ Mass – well defined
☐ Mass – poorly defined
☐ Spiculate mass
☐ Microcalcification
☐ Multifocal

Size .... mm

Distance from nipple ....mm

Co-ordinates ....

Left

☐ Asymmetry
☐ Distortion
☐ Mass – well defined
☐ Mass – poorly defined
☐ Spiculate mass
☐ Microcalcification
☐ Multifocal

Size .... mm

Distance from nipple ....mm

Co-ordinates ....

ULTRASOUND

Right   **Left**

Lesion Size .... mm   Lesion Size .... mm

Multifocal ....   Multifocal ....

P	1	2	3	4	5	P	1	2	3	4	5
M	1	2	3	4	5	M	1	2	3	4	5
U	1	2	3	4	5	U	1	2	3	4	5

BIOPSY   Consented Y/N

Right Side:

    US / STEREO

    FNA / Core Biopsy / VAB / Excision

    No of samples taken ....

    FNA Axilla   Y / N

    VAB Clip   Y / N

    MCC in spec No/ few/ mod/ abundant

Left Side:

    US / STEREO

    FNA / Core Biopsy / VAB / Excision

    No of samples taken ....

    FNA Axilla   Y / N

    VAB Clip   Y / N

    MCC in spec No/ few/ mod/ abundant

Comments:

> **Pathology to complete this box on receipt of specimen:**
> Specimen in pot – PRESENT OR ABSENT (Pls circle as appropriate.)

Issue No: 5   File Name: Assessment Biopsy Form V5 25.07.2017   Authorised by: QMSG
Review Date: August

Fig. 2.1 An example of a request form that can be used for core biopsies and fine needle aspirates

this is sufficient for making the diagnosis. Further sections are cut and examined if calcification was seen in the cores by the radiologist but has not been detected in the original sections. In a study of 168 cases of core biopsies with mammographic calcification, routine examination of 3 levels detected the calcification microscopically in 112 (67%) cases. Further sectioning (up to 10 sections) of 50 of the remaining cases, yielded calcification in 21 cases (42%). Out of these 21 cases, the diagnosis was changed in 11 cases (22%) after examining the new sections [4]. If the specimen x-ray was sent with the cores it is important to make sure that the calcifications in the sections correspond to those present in the x-ray. Very fine microcalcifications (less than 100 μm in diameter) which are sometimes detected in sections, are unlikely to be the ones seen in a mammogram; as the latter are usually coarser than that [5]. Lastly, it should be remembered that calcium oxalate crystals (Weddelite) do not stain with haematoxylin and can be easily missed during microscopic examination [6]. They usually appear as unstained faintly refractile crystals which are birefringent with polarised light. They are commonly present within relatively large benign cysts lined by apocrine epithelium [7, 8], and are seen only very rarely in association with DCIS [9].

The laboratory staff should be engaged in the process and understand the importance of their work. Good collaboration between the Laboratory staff and the pathologist are essential to guarantee getting timely, high quality, good stained sections that can be used in reaching the correct diagnosis.

The Pathologist

The diagnostic process starts by checking the patient's name and the case number, followed by reading the clinical and radiological information provided. The number of cores in the slide is compared with the number noted in the request form and in the Lab. It is important to remember that cores can sometime fragment during processing. A look at the stained sections by the naked eye can sometimes provide an idea about what to expect to see under the microscope. This also helps identifying where the cores are on the

slide, ensuring that on using the microscope all cores and fragments are examined.

The pathologist then examines the sections carefully and
makes the diagnosis. The most important step is to decide whether
the lesion is benign, malignant or border-line. The lesion is then
named and given a 'B' score to convey a clear message to the
treating physician about the nature of the lesion and how it should
be managed (B refers to the use of a wide 'Bore' needle, compared with the C score used in Cytology for fine needle aspirate).
The score extends from B1 to B5 as follows:

B1, Normal: indicates that the biopsy consists of normal breast
tissue or shows minimal changes like fibrosis, mildly dilated ducts
or minimal fine microcalcification. If these microscopic findings
do not correspond to the radiological ones, further sections may
have to be cut and if they are still negative, a repeat biopsy would
be indicated.

B2, Benign: A specific benign diagnosis can be made that cor-
responds to the radiologic findings. This would include lesions
like fibroadenoma, fibrocystic, fibroadenomatoid and columnar
cell change, benign cyst, sclerosing adenosis, duct ectasia, peri-
ductal mastitis, granulomatous mastitis, abscess, fat necrosis or
post-operative scars. These are usually lesions that do not need
surgical intervention.

B3, Benign with uncertain malignant potential: These are lesions
that are known to be sometimes associated with the presence of
malignancy or with a high risk of developing malignancy in the
future. Examples include Atypical intraductal epithelial proliferations (atypical ductal hyperplasia), flat epithelial atypia, in situ lobular neoplasia, benign or atypical papillary lesions, microglandular
adenosis, cellular fibroepithelial lesions, all non-malignant spindle
cell lesions, granular cell tumours and complex sclerosing lesions.
These lesions will usually need further clinical intervention in the
form of vacuum-associated needle excision or surgical excision.

B4, Suspicious, probably malignant: These are core biopsies
where there are a few atypical cells most likely malignant, but
their number is too small, or their morphology is markedly
distorted by crush artefact hindering a definite diagnosis of malignancy. A repeat biopsy is usually indicated in such cases.

B5, Malignant: Malignant cells are present in the core. This is subdivided into B5a for in situ carcinomas and B5b for invasive tumours whether they are carcinomas, sarcomas, malignant phyllodes or lymphomas.

The Multi-disciplinary Team Meeting (MDT)

All cases have to be then discussed in a multi-disciplinary meeting in the presence of Radiologists, Surgeons, Oncologists, Pathologists and Breast Care nurses. The clinical, radiological and pathological findings are presented and compared. If there are discrepancies a re-biopsy may have to be carried out. If the diagnosis is agreed, a plan is drawn for treatment (or no treatment in B2 cases). The Pathologist role in the meeting is essential and there should be facilities in the MDT room for projecting pictures of the cases under discussion, particularly for border-line lesions and for cases with unexpected findings.

References

1. Liberman L, Evans WP III, Dershaw DD, Hann LE, Deutch BM, Abramson AF, Rosen PP. Radiography of microcalcifications in stereotaxic mammary core biopsy specimens. Radiology. 1994;190:223–5.
2. Liberman L, Dershaw DD, Rosen PP, Abramson AF, Deutch BM, Hann LE. Stereotaxic 14-gauge breast biopsy: how many core biopsy specimens are needed. Radiology. 1994;192:793–5.
3. Philpotts LE, Shaheen NA, Carter D, Lange RC, Lee CH. Comparison of rebiopsy rates after stereotactic core needle biopsy of the breast with 11-gauge vacuum suction probe versus 14-gauge needle and automatic gun. AJR. 1999;172:683–7.
4. Grimes MM, Karageorge LS, Hogge JP. Does exhaustive search for microcalcifications improve diagnostic yield in stereotactic core needle breast biopsies? Mod Pathol. 2001;14:350–3.
5. Dahlstrom JE, Sutton S, Jain S. Histologic-radiologic correlation of mammographically detected microcalcification in stereotactic core biopsies. Am J Surg Pathol. 1998;22:256–9.
6. Tornos C, Silva E, El-Naggar A, Pritzker KPH. Calcium oxalate crystals in breast biopsies. The missing microcalcifications. Am J Surg Pathol. 1990;14:961–8.

7. Gonzalez JEG, Caldwell RG, Valaitis J. Calcium oxalate crystals in the breast. Pathology and significance. Am J Surg Pathol. 1991;15:586–91.
8. Truong LD, Cartwright J Jr, Alpert L. Calcium oxalate in breast lesions biopsied for calcification detected in screening mammography: incidence and clinical significance. Mod Pathol. 1992;5:146–52.
9. Singh N, Theaker JM. Calcium oxalate crystals (Weddellite) within the secretions of ductal carcinoma *in situ*—a rare phenomenon. J Clin Pathol. 1999;52:143–5.

Reporting Core Biopsies: Benign (B2) Lesions

3

Introduction: Is the Lesion Benign or Malignant?

This is the most important question the pathologist is required to answer. In most cases, a straightforward answer can be easily made once the slides have been examined. However, there are certain benign conditions that can be confused with malignancy, e.g. microglandular adenosis, extensive sclerosing adenosis and entrapped glands in the centre of a radial scar. It has to be noted here that the latter two lesions may be associated with smaller malignant elements. There are also border-line lesions where a benign or a malignant decision cannot be easily agreed upon. These include the atypical intraductal proliferative lesions, atypical apocrine lesions and atypical vascular lesions developing in the skin or breast tissue following radiotherapy. However, strict adherence to the standardised criteria for the diagnosis of these lesions can markedly reduce inter-observer disagreements [1].

Benign Lesions That Do Not Usually Need Further Intervention (B2 Lesions)

Fibroadenoma

Fibroadenomas are probably the most common benign lesions seen in core biopsies. They present mostly in young women in their late teens and twenties, although with the introduction of

© Springer Nature Switzerland AG 2020
S. Shousha, *Breast Pathology in Clinical Practice*, In Clinical Practice, https://doi.org/10.1007/978-3-030-42386-5_3

mammographic screening they are also being diagnosed now in much older women. They are usually single lesions that vary widely in size. In a review of 396 cases from Holland in females varying in age between 12 and 81 years (mean 33), the size varied between 1 and 220 mm [2]. In that study, 8% of the patients had multiple tumours that were bilateral in 3%.

In its usual form a fibroadenoma consists of bland hypocellular fibrous tissue and distorted glandular structures. Classically, two microscopic types are described, with no difference in behaviour: peri-canalicular, where the stroma surround the glandular elements (Fig. 3.1), and intra-canalicular (Fig. 3.2) where the epithelial elements are stretched out and the stroma may appear enclosed by the glands. Clefts may occur in the latter form making them confused with phyllodes tumours, but they lack the stromal hypercellularity characteristic of phyllodes tumours. However, recent research suggested the presence of similar gene mutation (recurrent *MED*12 exon 2) in juvenile intracanalicular fibroadenoma and benign phyllodes tumours [3].

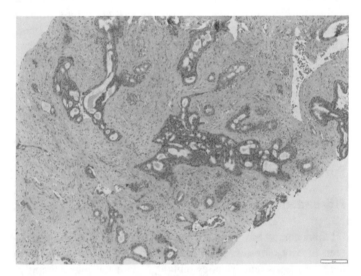

Fig. 3.1 Peri-canalicular fibroadenoma with usual type epithelial hyperplasia

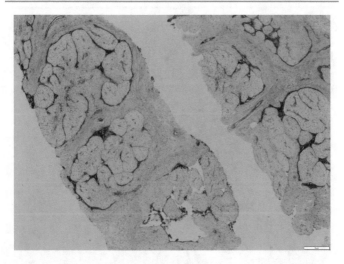

Fig. 3.2 Intracanalicular fibroadenoma

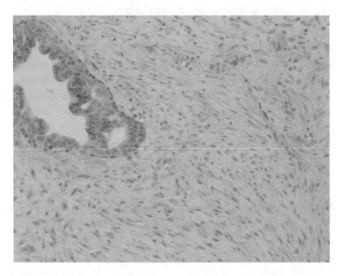

Fig. 3.3 Juvenile fibroadenoma with a mildly hypercellular stroma

A degree of stromal Hypercellularity may occur particularly in young girls, hence the name juvenile fibroadenoma (Fig. 3.3), but mitotic figures are absent or very rare (less than 1/10 high

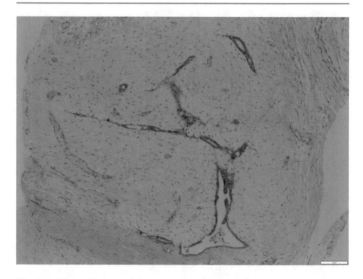

Fig. 3.4 Fibroadenoma with myxomatous change of the stroma

power field), except in pregnant women where an increase in mitotic activity may be seen. Myxomatous change of the stroma is not uncommon (Fig. 3.4), as well as areas of pseudoangiomatous hyperplasia. Osteoclast-type giant cells are occasionally seen in the stroma. In older women the stroma becomes hyalinised and focal calcification may occur (Fig. 3.5), leading to detection by radiology that is usually followed by a core biopsy. Columnar cell change of the epithelium is sometimes seen, and squamous metaplasia of the epithelium may be rarely present [2, 4]. Rarely infarctions may occur particularly during pregnancy and lactation or following biopsy procedure. A core biopsy of a fibroadenoma with any of the above changes is still scored as B2.

Epithelial hyperplasia, regular (Fig. 3.1) or atypical, may be also present, and very rarely foci of carcinoma in situ, ductal or lobular, are seen. In the above-mentioned review of 396 cases, ductal hyperplasia was present in 44%. This was mild in 12%, moderate in 27%, florid in 5% and atypical in 0.3% (one case).

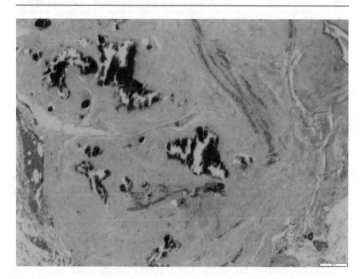

Fig. 3.5 Calcified fibroadenoma

Carcinoma in situ (five ductal and three lobular) was present in 2% of cases [2]. In another study of 2458 fibroadenomas, atypical ductal or lobular hyperplasia was present in 0.8% of cases, and on follow up, this did not seem to be associated with an increased risk of malignancy [5]. The presence of atypia within a fibroadenoma did not predict the presence of atypia in the adjacent breast tissue [5].

A study of 105 cases of carcinomas arising in fibroadenomas in patients varying in age between 15 and 83 years, showed that 90% of these were in situ tumours, with ductal and lobular type occurring with equal frequency and sometimes simultaneously [6]. Twenty one percent of these cases also had in situ carcinoma in the adjacent breast tissue. In that series 7% of the tumours were invasive ductal, and 3% invasive lobular, with 30% of these patients having invasive carcinoma in the adjacent breast tissue.

A core biopsy of a fibroadenoma with atypical hyperplasia is scored as B3 and those with in situ or invasive carcinoma are given a score of B5a and B5b respectively. These lesions will need surgical intervention, in contrast to the usual fibroadenomas, where surgery is not usually performed for lesions less than 3 cm in diameter.

Special Types of Fibroadenomas

Complex fibroadenoma: This is a concept which was introduced by Dupont et al. In 1994 to indicate a subgroup of fibroadenomas associated with a relative increased risk (×3.1) of developing breast carcinoma [7]. The lesion is defined as fibroadenomas with cysts greater than 3 mm in diameter, sclerosing adenosis, epithelial calcifications or papillary apocrine change (Fig. 3.6). The adjacent breast tissue may show proliferative fibrocystic change. Dupont' study included 2458 fibroadenomas, of which 558 (23%) were complex. Cysts only were present in 7%, papillary apocrine change in 4%, sclerosing adenosis in 3%, epithelial calcification in 1% and two or more features in the remaining 8%. Proliferative fibrocystic change was present in 18% of cases (compared with 12% in non-complex cases) including 2.3% with atypical hyperplasia (compared with 1.5% of non-complex cases). Cancer risk increases to 3.7 if there is a

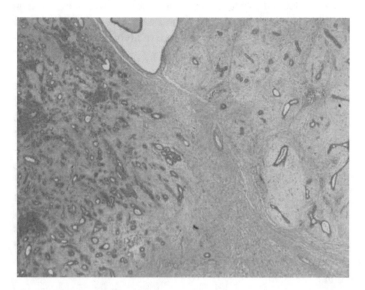

Fig. 3.6 Complex fibroadenoma with cysts and areas of sclerosing adenosis

family history of breast carcinoma (compared with a control group of patients with family history of breast cancer), and to 3.9 if there is adjacent proliferative fibrocystic change. In contrast, the same study found that patients with the usual type of fibroadenoma and no family history of breast cancer (two thirds of the studied cases) had no increased risk of developing carcinoma (1.08). The incidence of complex fibroadenoma in the Dutch study was 40%, was more common in older patients (mean age 35 years), and showed no relation to hyperplasia of adjacent tissue [2].

Lactational adenoma: Most of these lesions actually present during pregnancy as localised lumps, clinically resembling fibroadenomas. Microscopically, they consist of closely packed acinar structures, some could be cystic, with little intervening stroma. The cells show 'lactational change' in the form of vacuolated cytoplasm. Radiologically, it is a well-defined lesion. This helps in identifying it as an adenoma as histologically, in a core biopsy, it might look similar to normal lactational breast tissue.

'Lactational change' can be seen as a focal change in acini of non-pregnant, non-lactating women, usually in association with fibrocystic change. Many have a history of hormonal, antipsychotic or anti-hypertensive medications [8].

Tubular adenoma: A variant of pericanalicular fibroadenoma, where the glandular structures are numerous, mostly small and rounded, closely packed, and are separated by scanty fibrous tissue. Lesions composed partly of fibroadenoma and partly of tubular adenoma are sometimes seen; and combined tubular adenoma/tubular adenomyoepithelioma has been encountered. They tend to be softer than fibroadenomas [9].

Cellular fibroadenoma: This is a term used when there is mild to moderate increase in stromal cellularity. This is mostly observed in younger women.

Juvenile fibroadenoma (Fig. 3.3): This is a cellular fibroadenoma, usually with a peri-canalicular growth pattern, occurring in adolescents and young women. In addition to the stromal hypercellularity, epithelial gynaecomastoid/micropapillary usual type hyperplasia may be also present. Mitotic figures may be seen, usually not more than 2/10HPF, but can be as high as 6 or 7 particularly in lesions developing during pregnancy.

Recurrent fibroadenomas: In a study of 56 patients who had fibroadenomas at the age of 13–35 years, 14 (25%) reported the development of one or more additional fibroadenomas after the initial excision. Some patients had the recurrence at the previous excision site [10].

Fibroadenomatoid Change: This is a situation where relatively small localised areas in the core biopsy show features similar to those seen in fibroadenoma, i.e. haphazardly arranged glandular elements in a stroma different from that seen in the adjacent normal breast tissue, but they lack the well-circumscribed mass outline seen, radiologically and histologically, in a fibroadenoma (Fig. 3.7).

Hamartoma

This is one of the most difficult diagnosis to make in a core biopsy. Breast hamartomas consist of normal breast elements that are arranged in a haphazard manner. They differ from fibroadenomas by containing additional benign elements in beside the

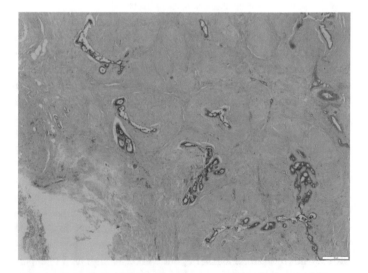

Fig. 3.7 Focal fibroadenomatoid change

glands and fibrous tissue. The commonest additional element is fat. Radiologically a hamartoma appears as a well-defined lesion like a fibroadenoma, but may show a heterogeneous echogenicity due to the presence of fat. A core biopsy will show a mixture of normal breast elements, including at most some mildly dilated glands, and the core will usually be given a score of B1 indicating normal breast tissue. If the lesion is of a small size, it is usually left behind with no need for surgery. In the rare case where the lesion is big enough to necessitate removal, the real nature of the lesion can be realised by the pathologist.

Myoid hamartoma is a rare form of breast hamartome where the stroma consists of myoid elements that stain positively for smooth muscle immune stains like SMA and Desmin. In H&E stained sections the lesion consists of scattered small glands and a spindle cell stroma that resembles, to some extent, smooth muscle fibres which leads the pathologist to stain for smooth muscle fibres, hence the right diagnosis is reached and a score of B2 is given to the core (Fig. 3.8). Foci of sclerosing adenosis are sometimes seen at the edge of the lesion.

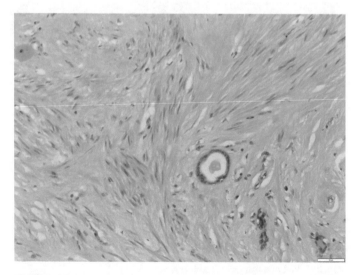

Fig. 3.8 Myoid hamartoma. Bundles of spindle shaped cells with interspersed glands

Fibrocystic Change

These are probably the second most common group of benign (B2) lesions diagnosed in core biopsies that do not need further treatment. The patients are usually in their reproductive period of life.

The simplest form is a benign cyst, which can be a large single cyst detected by radiology, lined by simple cuboidal epithelium surrounded by fibrous tissue. The diagnosis can be made by finding parts of the cyst wall in the core biopsy (Fig. 3.9). Sometimes, if the cyst was traumatised before the biopsy is taken, evidence of cyst rupture is seen in the form of an inflammatory reaction composed of foamy histiocytes and lymphocytes (Fig. 3.10).

The term fibrocystic change is usually used when there are other elements in addition to the presence of scattered cysts of variable, but mostly microscopic, sizes (Fig. 3.11). Prominent microcalcification may be present (Fig. 3.12). The cysts can be

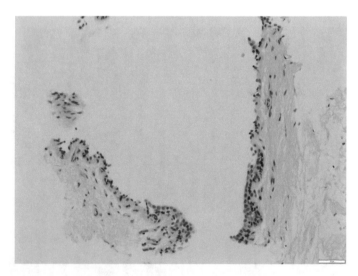

Fig. 3.9 Part of a benign cyst wall in a core biopsy

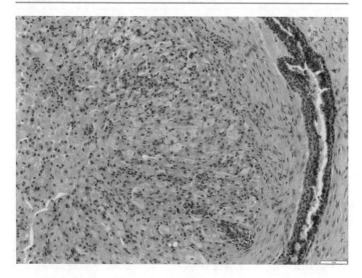

Fig. 3.10 Inflammatory reaction rich in foamy histiocytes indicating a ruptured cyst

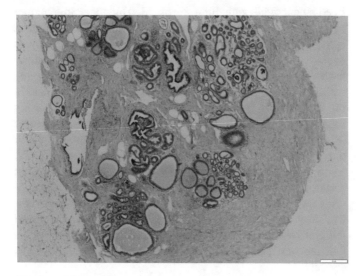

Fig. 3.11 Fibrocystic change

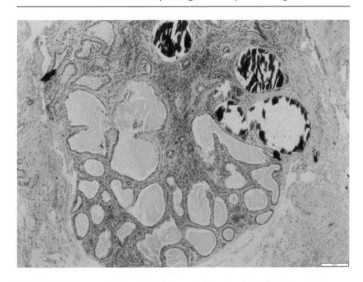

Fig. 3.12 Fibrocystic change with prominent microcalcification

lined by cuboidal epithelium, surrounded by myoepithelium, or
by apocrine type epithelium that has abundant pink stained
cytoplasm and small nuclei (Fig. 3.13). Apocrine cysts may be
devoid of myoepithelium, and may show complex papillary
proliferations. There may be also foci of adenosis. These are
well-defined areas of proliferating small terminal ductules. In
the simple form the glands remain intact and distinct, being
separated from each other by minimal fibrous tissue stroma
(Fig. 3.14). Lymphocytic infiltration may be present. In spite of
the name, excess fibrous tissue is not a common feature.
Microcalcification, in the form of dark blue-stained foci within
glands or stroma, may be present but not commonly so. In apocrine cysts calcification is usually in the form of calcium oxalate crystals which in H&E stained sections remain unstained
but can be detected as vaguely perceptible retractile crystals
that are best seen by polarising microscopy as birefrengent
crystals.

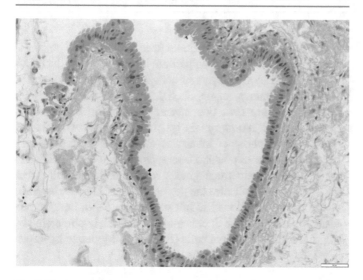

Fig. 3.13 Apocrine cyst

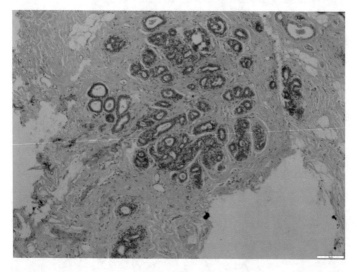

Fig. 3.14 Focal adenosis

Ductal Hyperplasia

Another feature that is commonly seen in fibrocystic change is hyperplasia of the ductal epithelium. Normal breast ducts and acini are lined by two layers of cells, an inner epithelial and an outer, discontinuous, myoepithelial. Hyperplasia indicates the presence of more than two layers. Hyperplasia of mammary ducts is divided into two main types: regular or usual type and atypical. Hyperplasia of lobules is always considered atypical and will be considered later. Usual type ductal hyperplasia is further subdivided into three grades: mild, moderate and florid. Mild hyperplasia indicates the presence of three or four layers of cells in the duct wall instead of two (Fig. 3.15). In florid hyperplasia, the lumen of the duct is almost completely obliterated by the proliferating epithelial cells (Fig. 3.16). Moderate hyperplasia is intermediate between the two.

Differentiating Regular Hyperplasia (B2) from Atypical Hyperplasia (B3) and Low Grade DCIS (B5a)

It is important to distinguish florid regular hyperplasia from atypical hyperplasia and low grade DCIS. In florid regular hyperpla-

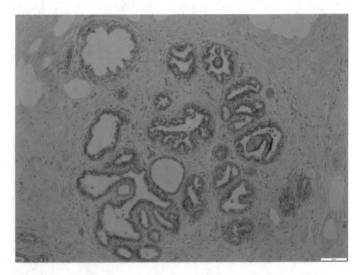

Fig. 3.15 Mild usual type ductal hyperplasia in a focus of adenosis

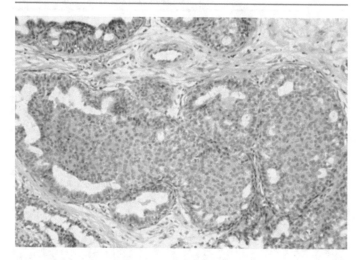

Fig. 3.16 Florid usual type ductal hyperplasia

sia, the proliferating cells are similar to the normal cells lining the ducts with no evidence of nuclear atypia or central necrosis. Myoepithelial cells with spindle shaped nuclei are usually seen interspersed between the epithelial cells. The hyperplastic cells may assume a streaming pattern and irregular peripheral, and central, lumina may be present (Figs. 3.16 and 3.17).

In atypical ductal hyperplasia, there are cytological and architectural abnormalities which are usually limited to a group of cells within the involved duct, with the peripheral cells, at least in part of the duct, remaining normal in shape and polarisation (Fig. 3.18). Cytologically, there is a variable degree of nuclear pleomorphism and hyperchromasia (which can be classified as mild, moderate or severe). Architecturally, low papillary, cribriform or 'Roman bridges' patterns may be present [11, 12]. Atypical hyperplasia on its own is relatively uncommon. It is more commonly seen around or near malignant lesions. Its presence in a core biopsy should arouse the suspicion of a nearby carcinoma, and more sections have to be examined. Many cases with atypical hyperplasia on core biopsies (up to 50% in some studies), will show carcinoma, in situ or invasive, on excision [13, 14]. Features predictive of upgrade include the presence of a radiological lesion, the extent

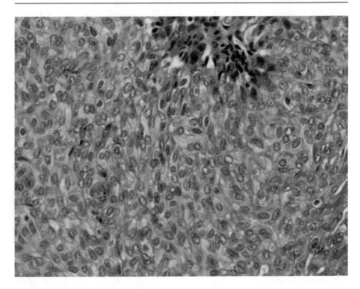

Fig. 3.17 Florid usual type ductal hyperplasia. High power view showing cellular streaming

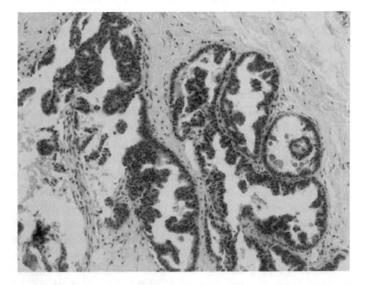

Fig. 3.18 Atypical ductal hyperplasia

and number of cores showing atypical hyperplasia and older patient age [14]. In a study of 110 patients with atypical ductal hyperplasia on core biopsy, 40% had DCIS on excision which was associated with invasive carcinoma in 8%. All invasive lesions were 8 mm or less, ER positive, axillary node negative. Two were HER2 positive [13].

In contrast to atypical ductal hyperplasia, low grade DCIS is characterised by a monomorphic cell population, in two ducts at least, or scattered over an area less than 2 mm, with no intermingled spindle myoepithelial cells. The cribriform spaces, when present in DCIS, are geometrically regular and rounded. If only one duct is involved or the changes occupy an area less than 2 mm, the case is considered atypical hyperplasia provided the biopsy has been thoroughly sampled.

When the hyperplasia is extensive causing marked expansion of the involved duct, differentiating it from low grade DCIS may be difficult in H& E stained sections. In this situation immunostaining for CK5 or CK5/6 or ER (Fig. 3.19c) is helpful. Usual

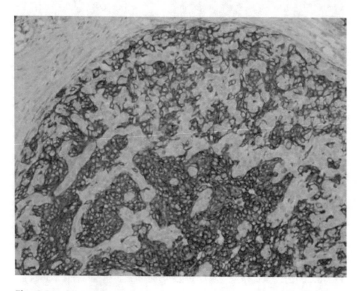

Fig. 3.19 CK5 staining of florid usual type ductal hyperplasia showing a mosaic pattern of staining

type hyperplasia, being a mixture of proliferating luminal (CK5 negative/ER positive) and myoepithelial (CK5 positive/ER negative) cells, will give rise to a mosaic pattern of staining composed of mixed positive and negative cells (Figs. 3.19 and 3.20). In most DCIS, all the proliferating neoplastic cells are CK5 negative, although occasional one or two positive cells may be present. In atypical hyperplasia, the atypical cells grouped in part of the involved ducts would be CK5 negative [12].

Columnar Cell Change and Columnar Cell Hyperplasia

Columnar cell change is a relatively common benign condition which may be seen on its own or in association with fibrocystic change. It involves individual lobules leading to dilatation of the

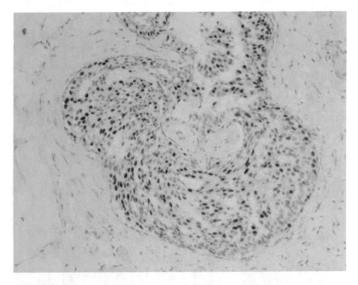

Fig. 3.20 ER staining of florid usual type ductal hyperplasia showing a mosaic pattern

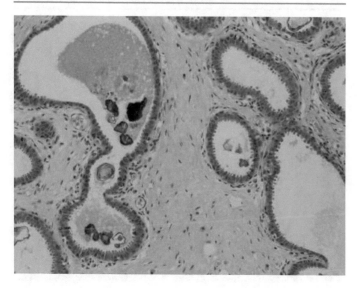

Fig. 3.21 Columnar cell change with luminal calcification

acini which become lined by a layer of simple columnar epithelium with elongated nuclei, arranged perpendicular to the basement membrane with no evidence of atypia. The cells have prominent apical 'snouts' that protrude into the glandular lumen which commonly contains eosinophilic secretion (Fig. 3.21). Luminal microcalcification is common leading to their mammographic detection. The columnar cells are ER strongly and uniformly positive (Fig. 3.22) and CK5 negative (Fig. 3.23). The lesions can be multifocal and usually occur in women 35–50 year old.

In columnar cell hyperplasia (Fig. 3.24), the dilated glands are lined by more than one layer of columnar cells which retain their benign features with no evidence of atypia or architectural complexity. The presence of architectural complexity, in the form of tufts, Roman bridges, micropapillary or cribriform patterns (Fig. 3.24) is usually associated with a degree of nuclear atypia which would justify moving the lesion into the category of atypical ductal hyperplasia (B3).

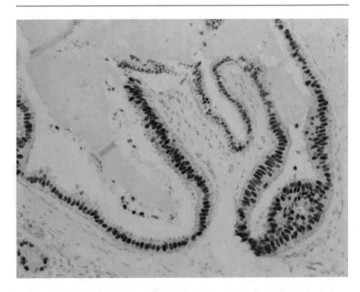

Fig. 3.22 Columnar cell change. Strong diffuse staining for ER

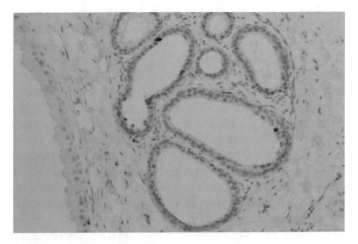

Fig. 3.23 Columnar cell change. Negative CK5 staining

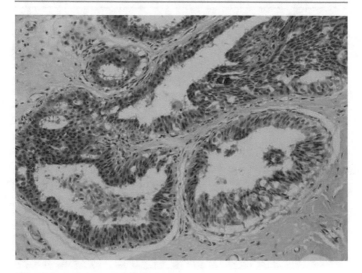

Fig. 3.24 Columnar cell hyperplasia

Sclerosing Adenosis and Apocrine Adenosis

In contrast to adenosis, as described above as part of fibrocystic change, in sclerosing adenosis, the involved lobule remains well defined but the central glands appear compressed, loosing their lumina and are separated by proliferating myofibroblasts (Fig. 3.25). The peripheral glands may appear dilated. The size of each focus remains microscopic, but sometimes large foci may occur and in rare cases there may be large multiple closely backed foci, that can produce palpable hard lump mimicking malignant tumours clinically. These are sometimes called 'adenosis tumours' (Fig. 3.26).

Apocrine adenosis is a similar lesion in which the involved acini are lined by apocrine cells with abundant eosinophilic cytoplasm and small basal nuclei (Fig. 3.27). Atypia or in situ malignant change may affect both lesions, in which case such cores would be scored as B3 or B5a respectively.

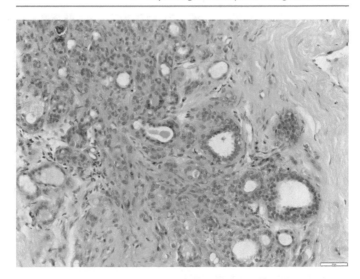

Fig. 3.25 Sclerosing adenosis

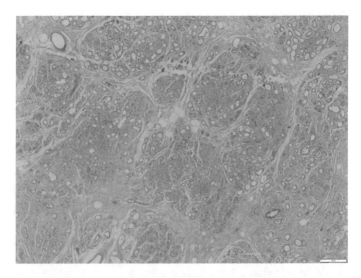

Fig. 3.26 Nodular sclerosing adenosis (adenosis tumour)

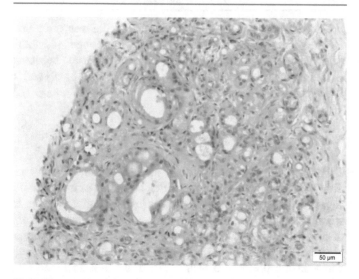

50 μm

Fig. 3.27 Apocrine adenosis

Duct Ectasia

This is one of the most over-diagnosed breast lesions. The presence of one or a few slightly dilated ducts is not an uncommon incidental finding in breast biopsies, and a degree of ductal dilatation is commonly seen in association with other lesions particularly intraduct papillomas. In true duct ectasia, the dilated ducts are distended with thick secretion and are usually easily seen by the naked eye in the gross specimen. Microscopically, the markedly dilated ducts contain inspissated secretion and are surrounded by heavy lymphocytic infiltration and fibrosis. The ducts are usually irregular in outline and are lined by cuboidal epithelium which may be atrophic in some areas, or may occasionally show a degree of hyperplasia. The intervening stroma may be also inflamed, and cholesterol granulomas are sometimes present. In later stages, inflammation may subside and the ducts become surrounded by dense fibrous tissue. Some cases, up to 47% in one series [15] are associated with high serum

prolactin levels, which occasionally may be the result of a prolactin producing pituitary adenoma [16] or prolonged phenothiazine therapy [17]. The age incidence is 30–80 years, but it has
also been described in male and female children [18, 19] and in
adult males [20].

Granulomatous Mastitis

Granulomatous lobular mastitis is an inflammatory breast condition of unclear aetiology, for which hormonal or autoimmune
causes have been suggested [21]. The lesion usually develops in
women in their reproductive age with a relatively recent history
of pregnancy. In a published series of 87 women, the average
age was 35 years and 63% of patients had a history of pregnancy in the previous 5 years [21]. The series included four
additional men who had the disease. The lesion presents clinically as a painful irregular hard lump that can be mistaken for
carcinoma. The correct diagnosis is usually reached by examination of a core biopsy. Microscopically, there is heavy infiltration of the breast tissue with chronic inflammatory cells,
including occasional foreign body type giant cells, that have a
distinct lobular distribution surrounding injured ducts. No well-
formed granulomas are present and stains for organisms are
negative. Abscesses may develop in advanced cases. Currently,
the disease is managed conservatively with no need for surgical
intervention [21].

Cystic neutrophilic granulomatous mastitis is a more recently
described distinct entity of the disease in which a bacteriological
aetiology is suspected. The clinical presentation is similar to
granulomatous lobular mastitis. Microscopically, the core
biopsy shows well-defined rounded cystic spaces surrounded by
neutrophils with adjacent heavy infiltration with chronic inflammatory cells, which may include an occasional foreign body
type giant cell (Figs. 3.28 and 3.29) Gram positive bacilli, identified to be of *Corynebacterium* species have been isolated from
the lesions and can occasionally be seen within the cystic spaces

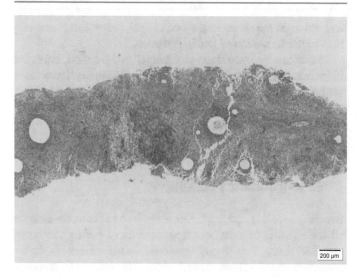

Fig. 3.28 Cystic neutrophilic granulomatous mastitis. Heavy inflammatory reaction and interspersed cystic spaces

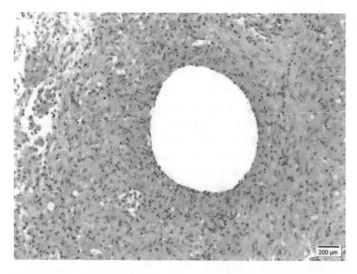

Fig. 3.29 Cystic neutrophilic granulomatous mastitis. High power view showing a cystic space surrounded by inflammatory cells rich in neutrophils

and amongst the inflammatory cells [22]. Advanced forms may lead to the formation of small abscesses.

Tuberculosis, sarcoidosis and fungal and parasitic infections (for example Schistosomiasis), could also lead to the formation of well-formed granulomas in the breast and should be included in the differential diagnosis. A foreign body giant cell reaction is sometimes seen around amyloid deposits in breast core biopsies in patients with amyloidosis.

Other Inflammatory Conditions

Breast abscesses are not uncommon and can develop in advanced cases of granulomatous mastitis, or during pregnancy and lactation. Peri-ductal mastitis, where there is heavy lymphocytic infiltration around ducts, can sometimes be symptomatic, leading to core biopsy. It is suspected to be more common in smokers.

Other Less Common Benign Conditions

Galactoceles are cysts containing milk that may develop during lactation. A core biopsy will show a cystic space containing structureless secretion surrounded by foamy histiocytes. The surrounding breast tissue shows evidence of lactational change.

Pseudo-lactational change can occur as small foci in association with fibrocystic change or in their own, and are characterised by the presence of acini lined by cuboidal cells with vacuolated cytoplasm and no nuclear atypia (Fig. 3.30). Cases with atypical hyperplasia do occur and would be scored as B3.

Haemangiomas may present radiologically as echogenic areas that lead to biopsy. The core will show multiple closely packed thin-walled vascular spaces full of red blood cells. Rare cases may develop after radiotherapy to the breast and have to be differentiated from angiosarcoma.

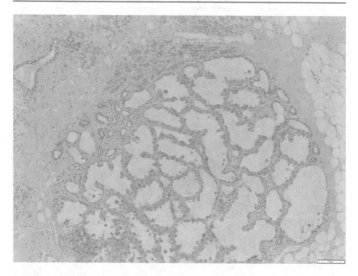

Fig. 3.30 Pseudo-lactational change

Lymphangiomas have been rarely seen in punch biopsies of the breast skin in previously irradiated areas.

Lipomas can present radiologically as well defined lesions that are usually biopsied. A core biopsy will show mature adipose tissue. As this cannot be differentiated from normal breast fat, a score of B1 is usually given with an additional statement in the text indicating that it would be consistent with lipoma.

Stromal coarse calcification, on the other hand, might be given a score of B2, when it is so prominent in a core biopsy carried out for radiological calcification with no evidence of any other abnormality in the core.

Diabetic Mastopathy presents as a hard lump in patients with type 2 diabetes mellitus, that can be clinically confused with carcinoma. A core biopsy will show dense fibrous tissue, that might include atypical myofibroblasts with enlarged nuclei, and scattered lymphocytic aggregates (Figs. 3.30 and 3.31).

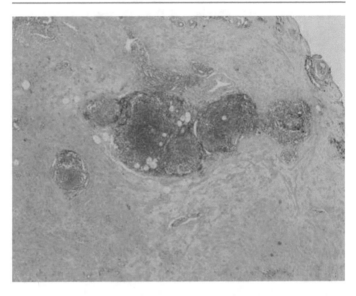

Fig. 3.31 Diabetic mastopathy. Dense fibrous stroma and prominent lymphocytic aggregates

References

1. Schnitt SJ, Connolly JL, Tavassoli FA, Fechner RE, Kempson RL, Gelman R, Page DL. Interobserver reproducibility in the diagnosis of ductal proliferative breast lesions using standardized criteria. Hum Pathol. 1992;16:1133–43.
2. Kuijper A, Mommers ECM, van der Wall E, van Diest PJ. Histopathology of fibroadenomas of the breast. Am J Clin Pathol. 2001;115:736–42.
3. Pareja F, Da Cruz Paula A, Murray MP, Hoang T, Gularte-Merida R, Brown D, et al. Recurrent *MED12* exon2 mutations in benign breast fibroepithelial lesions in adolescents and young adults. J Clin Pathol. 2019;72:258–62.
4. Shousha S. Squamous metaplasia in fibroadenomas of the breast. Histopathology. 1986;10:1001–2.
5. Carter BA, Page DL, Schuyler P, Parl FF, Simpson JF, Jensen RA, Dupont WD. No elevation in long-term breast carcinoma risk for women with fibroadenomas that contain atypical hyperplasia. Cancer. 2001;92:30–6.
6. Diaz NM, Palmer JO, McDivitt RW. Carcinoma arising within fibroadenomas of the breast. A clinicopathologic study of 105 patients. Am J Clin Pathol. 1991;95:614–22.

7. Dupont WD, Page DL, Parl FF, Vnencak-Jones CL, Plummer WD Jr, Rados MS, Schuyler PA. Long-term risk of breast cancer in women with fibroadenoma. N Engl J Med. 1994;331:10–5.
8. Tavassoli FA, Yeh IT. Lactational and clear cell changes of the breast in nonlactating, nonpregnant women. Am J Clin Pathol. 1987;87:23–9.
9. Hertel BF, Zaloudek C, Kempson RL. Breast adenomas. Cancer. 1976;37:2891–905.
10. Javid A, Jenkins SM, Labow B, Boughey JC, Lamaine V, Neal L, et al. Intermediate and long-term outcomes of fibroadenoma excision in adolescent and young adult patients. Breast J. 2019;25:91–5.
11. Page DL, Rogers LW. Combined histologic and cytologic criteria for the diagnosis of mammary atypical ductal hyperplasia. Hum Pathol. 1992;23:1095–7.
12. Quintana LM, Collins LC. Assessing intraductal proliferations in breast core needle biopsies. Diagn Histopathol. 2017;24:49–57.
13. Farshid G, Edwards S, Kollias J, Grantley GP. Active surveillance of women diagnosed with atypical ductal hyperplasia on core needle biopsy may spare many women potentially unnecessary surgery, but at the risk of undertreatment for a minority: 10-year surgical outcomes of 114 consecutive cases from a single center. Mod Pathol. 2018;31:395–405.
14. Salageen ED, Slodkowska E, Nofech-Mozes S, Hanna W, Para-Herran C, Lu F-I. Atypical ductal hyperplasia on core needle biopsy: development of a predictive model stratifying carcinoma upgrade risk on excision. Breast J. 2019;25:56–61.
15. Peters F, Schuth W. Hyperprolactinemia and nonpuerperal mastitis (duct ectasia). JAMA. 1989;261:1618–20.
16. Shousha S, Backhouse CM, Dawson PM, Alaghband-Zadeh J, Burn I. Mammary duct ectasia and pituitary adenomas. Am J Surg Pathol. 1988;12:130–3.
17. Hunter-Craig ID, Tuddenham EGD, Earle JHO. Lipogranuloma of the breast due to phenothiazine therapy. Br J Surg. 1970;57:76–9.
18. Stringel G, Perelman A, Jimenez C. Infantile mammary duct ectasia: a cause of bloody nipple discharge. J Pediatr Surg. 1986;21:671–4.
19. Miller JD, Brownell MD, Shaw A. Bilateral breast masses and bloody nipple discharge in a 4-year-old boy. J Pediatr. 1990;116:744–74.
20. Mansel RE, Morgan WP. Duct ectasia in the male. Br J Surg. 1979;66:660–2.
21. Berreto DS, Sedgwick EL, Nagi CS, Benveniste AP. Granulomatous mastitis: etiology, pathology, treatment, and clinical findings. Breast Cancer Res Treat. 2018;171:527–34.
22. Troxell ML, Gordon NT, Stone Dogett J, Ballard M, Vetto JT, Pommier RF, Naik AM. Cystic neutrophilic granulomatous mastitis. Association with Gram positive bacilli and Corynebacterium. Am J Clin Pathol. 2016;145:635–45.

Reporting Core Biopsies: Benign Lesions That Usually Need Further Intervention (B3 Lesions)

4

Introduction

This is the most difficult category in the spectrum of core biopsies. Difficult for the pathologist to make, for the treating physician to decide what to do and difficult for the patent to understand. For Pathologists distinction of these lesions from B2 lesions can be problematic (for example usual type hyperplasia from atypical hyperplasia, a cellular fibroadenoma from a phyllodes tumour or a columnar cell change from flat epithelial atypia). For the treating physician, In contrast to the other four categories where action is usually clear, the action here varies between follow up, vacuum excision or surgical excision and a decision has to be made. For patients, they commonly wonder and ask if they are benign why do I have to do an operation or another discomforting procedure? Hence it is important to stick to the up-to-date accepted criteria for diagnosis and guidelines for management and explain to the patient the reason for any action taken. Particularly as these lesions are usually discovered during routine mammographic screening, either as a result of microcalcification, distortion or 'echogenic' abnormality, in women who are complaining of nothing.

Indeed, B3 lesions are benign and many stay benign even after excision, but sometimes they hide sinister lesions behind them and the only way to detect these sinister lesions is by removing more surrounding tissue. Furthermore, one more of the same lesion sometimes changes the diagnosis: more than one atypical ductal hyperplasia changes the diagnosis to low grade ductal

© Springer Nature Switzerland AG 2020
S. Shousha, *Breast Pathology in Clinical Practice*, In Clinical Practice, https://doi.org/10.1007/978-3-030-42386-5_4

carcinoma in situ. Still other B3 lesions have no clear natural history and as we do not know how they would behave if left behind it is thought to be more advisable to remove them.

Atypical Epithelial Hyperplasia (ADH)

Distinguishing florid usual type ductal hyperplasia from atypical ductal hyperplasia has been discussed in Chap. 3 and illustrated in Figs. 3.16–3.20. The important thing to remember is that the presence of a few atypical cells in a hyperplastic lesion does not make it atypical. A reasonable part of the duct, or the whole of a single duct, should be involved by monomorphic low nuclear grade neoplastic cells that would stain negative for CK5 if this is done. If two separate ducts are involved or if the cells have intermediate or high grade nuclei, the lesion is considered DCIS. The second international consensus conference on breast lesions of uncertain malignant potential, recommends surgical excision of all lesions with atypical ductal hyperplasia diagnosed on core or vacuum biopsy [1].

Flat Epithelial Atypia (FEA)

This is a form of mammary epithelial atypia that has been relatively more recently described as it became more commonly detected, together with columnar cell change, as a result of routine mammographic screening, as both types of lesions are often associated with prominent microcalcification. The two lesions are not uncommonly seen together and are probably related as sometimes a single duct can be seen partly lined by columnar cells and partly by the cells characteristic of FEA. The calcification is present in the lumina of the involved ducts.

The cells of FEA are cuboidal, rather than columnar, and have characteristic rounded slightly enlarged darkly stained nuclei that show a mild degree of atypia and loss of polarity with some cells appearing as if they are lying on their sides rather than perpendicular to the basement membrane (Fig. 4.1). The lumen of

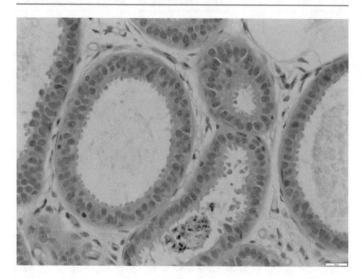

Fig. 4.1 Flat epithelial atypia. Note the rounded hyperchromatic mildly dysplastic nuclei and flat inner luminal surface

the duct is usually nicely rounded, rather than undulated as is usually seen in columnar cell change. However, more than one layer of cells may be present which may lead to an irregular luminal contour. If the lining cells start piling up to form humps, papillae or Roman bridges, the case is considered as atypical ductal hyperplasia rather than FEA (Figs. 4.2 and 4.3). The cells are strongly and uniformly ER positive (Fig. 4.4a) and CK5 negative (Fig. 4.4b), similar to columnar cell change. In contrast to ADH, the term FEA can be used even if several ducts are involved by the change. If the nuclear atypia is of a moderate or high grade, the case is considered as representing flat DCIS, of moderate or high grade.

FEA is considered benign but is known to be sometimes associated with neoplastic lesions particularly lobular neoplasia and tubular carcinoma. In a recent study from France, 3 (15%) out of 20 patients with pure FEA on vacuum biopsies (not associated with any other risk lesions) were upgraded to carcinoma; 1 low grade DCIS, 1 intermediate grade DCIS and 1 grade 2

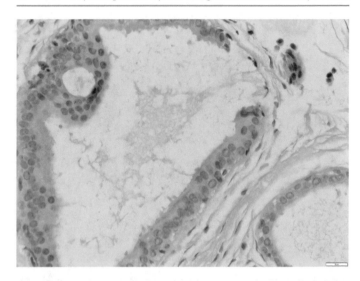

Fig. 4.2 Atypical ductal hyperplasia with a cribriform pattern arising on top of flat epithelial atypia

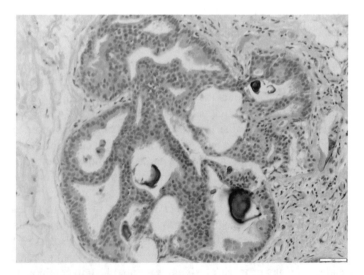

Fig. 4.3 Atypical ductal hyperplasia with complex architecture, arising on top of flat epithelial atypia. Note the presence of luminal microcalcification

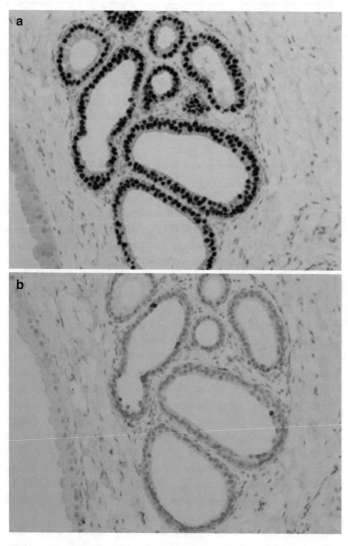

Fig. 4.4 Flat epithelial atypia: (**a**) ER strongly positive; (**b**) CK5 negative

invasive ductal carcinoma. Factors associated with upgrading included an age of 57 years or older, radiologic size more than 10 mm and the presence of four or more foci of FEA [2]. In a recent review and meta-analysis study, the upgrade of FEA to malignancy on excision was 11% [3]. It is recommended that cases of pure flat epithelial atypia (not associated with ADH) to be managed by vacuum excision followed by active surveillance [1].

In Situ Lobular Neoplasia

Normal breast lobules consist of a group of acini separated by minimal amount of specialised fibrous stroma. All normal epithelial cells of the breast, including those lining normal acini, show strong positive membrane expression of E-Cadherin. The appearance of cells lacking the expression of membrane E-Cadherin heralds the appearance of lobular neoplasia in these acini. In my opinion this is not a hyperplastic process as there are no normal E-cadherin negative cells from which they can proliferate. Also, it is not a metaplastic process as there are no equivalent normal cells anywhere in the breast. Many authors now consider it a neoplastic process reflecting a genetic abnormality involving the E-cadherin pathway, no matter how many E-cadherin negative cells are present or how many acini are involved. Originally, lobular lesions were divided into two types according to the percentage of acini involved in a given lobule. If the acini involved are less than 50% the process is called atypical lobular hyperplasia (ALH) and if more than 50% it is lobular carcinoma in situ (LCIS). Many authors now consider this distinction misleading, difficult to make, and could be alarming to patients by including the word carcinoma in some of these lesions which by themselves are mostly not life threatening. Hence all such lesions are now considered to represent in situ lobular neoplasia, as long as the surrounding basement membrane is intact. If the basement membrane is breached, they are invasive lobular carcinomas. It has to be added here, that in rare cases, the loss of E-cadherin expression is only partial and that in rare cases of invasive lobular carcinoma,

E-cadherin expression is preserved as a result of a particular genetic fault in its pathway.

So, the term atypical lobular hyperplasia can be easily abandoned and it has been abandoned by many authors. But, the term lobular carcinoma in situ (LCIS) still persists and it is very difficult to know where to draw the line between in situ lobular neoplasia and LCIS. Perhaps the term LCIS should be restricted to the pleomorphic variant (see below).

The acini in in situ lobular neoplasia appear distended with uniform, monomorphic, small or medium sized rounded neoplastic cells with uniformly rounded dark-stained nuclei. A degree of cellular dis-cohesion is typical of this lesion (Fig. 4.5a). Mucin may be present in the cytoplasm. The involved acini may become enlarged and distorted. Immunostaining for E-Cadherin is mostly negative (Fig. 4.5b), ER is strongly positive (Fig. 4.5c) and CK5 negative. Microcalcification is not usually present, but may be seen in occasions (Fig. 4.6). Cases have been classified according to the nuclear size of the tumour cells and the number of lobules involved, as discussed below.

In core biopsies, in situ lobular neoplasia may be encountered in several situations. The simplest form is a few involved acini found incidentally in a biopsy carried out for a different lesion, for example a fibroadenoma. The fibroadenoma is present in the core biopsy with a few adjacent acini showing minor involvement with in situ lobular neoplasia (Fig. 4.6). This is a situation where B3 would be justified but the management can vary between follow up observation or a vacuum excision. With the presence of more abundant involved acini, a vacuum excision may be strongly recommended [1]. There is a third less common situation where the whole core is occupied with closely packed foci of in situ lobular neoplasia (Fig. 4.7). The first impression on examining such a core would be of a low grade DCIS, but the morphology of the cells as described above hints at the possibility of in situ lobular neoplasia, a diagnosis which is confirmed by negative E-Cadherin staining (Fig. 4.7). The condition is sometimes called 'florid in situ lobular neoplasia' and the recommendation now is to give such a lesion a score of B5a with recommendation for surgical excision [1]. In a further

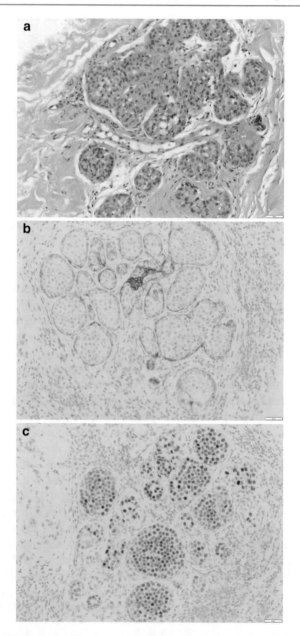

Fig. 4.5 In situ lobular neoplasia: (**a**) H&E; (**b**) Negative E-Cadherin membrane staining; (**c**) Positive ER nuclear staining

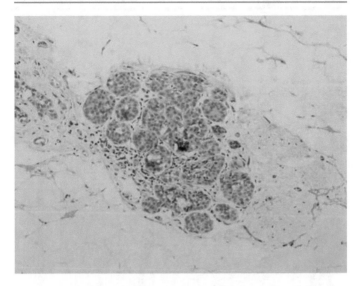

Fig. 4.6 An incidental focus of in situ lobular neoplasia with microcalcification, seen in a core biopsy beside a fibroadenoma

situation in situ lobular neoplasia may be seen in association with DCIS, hence a B5a would be given In this context it may be worth mentioning that it is not uncommon to see marked proliferation of myoepithelial cells around or within foci of in situ lobular neoplasia (Fig. 4.8). These proliferating myoepithelial cells lack atypia, stain positivity with myoepithelial markers, and these lesions should not be confused with combined in situ lobular neoplasia/DCIS [4, 5]. A last least common situation in which in situ lobular neoplasia is encountered in a core biopsy is when the lobular cells have the same characteristic as described above except for the fact they have large pleomorphic nuclei leading to what is called pleomorphic LCIS (Fig. 4.9). These cases can be easily confused with high grade DCIS. Indeed comedo necrosis and microcalcification may be present. These cases are given a B5a score with a recommended surgical excision [1]. Many cases prove on excision to have associated invasive lobular carcinoma. It has to be added here that the presence of microcalcification is sometimes seen in the other simpler forms described above and should not be a cause for upgrading the score to B4 or B5.

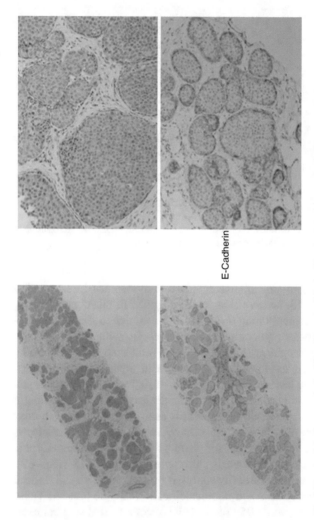

E-Cadherin

Fig. 4.7 Florid in situ lobular neoplasia. Closely packed foci of in situ lobular neoplasia. Top raw H&E low and high power views. Bottom raw: E-Cadherin negative staining: low and high power views

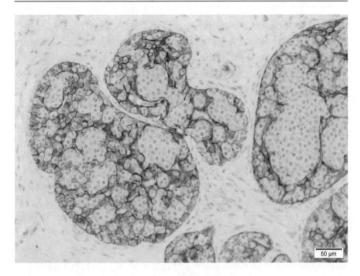

Fig. 4.8 E-Cadherin staining of foci of in situ lobular neoplasia (E-cadherin negative) with marked proliferation of myoepithelial cells (E-cadherin positive and also positive for myoepithelial markers—not shown)

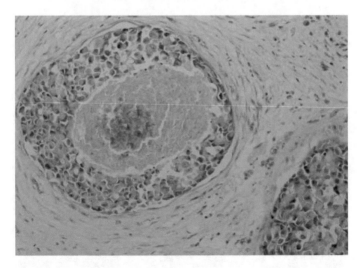

Fig. 4.9 Pleomorphic in situ lobular neoplasia/lobular carcinoma in situ, with comedo necrosis and central calcification. Note the presence of cellular in-cohesion with large pleomorphic nuclei

The reported rates of conversion of in situ lobular neoplasia in core biopsies to more advanced lesions on excision varies between 12 and 22% according to the type and extent of the lesion [3]. This rises to 36% in pleomorphic LCIS [6].

Radial Scar/Complex Sclerosing Lesions

These are uncommon lesions that are usually detected as mammographic distortion or small stellate lesions that can be easily confused radiologically and microscopically with small invasive carcinomas. Lesions measuring less than 10 mm are called radial scars and the larger ones are called complex sclerosing lesions, but the basic structures are the same. In a core biopsy the diagnostic feature is the presence of an area of fibroelastosis in which distorted glands are embedded, surrounded by a variety of proliferative epithelial lesions including cysts, adenosis, sclerosing adenosis, apocrine metaplasia, usual type ductal hyperplasia and small benign intraduct papillomas (Fig. 4.10). The distorted

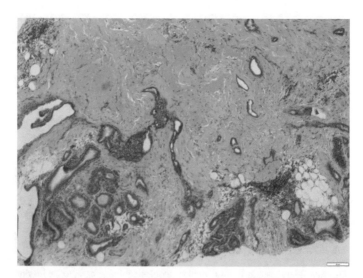

Fig. 4.10 Radial scar with a fibro-elastotic centre surrounded by proliferating epithelia cells

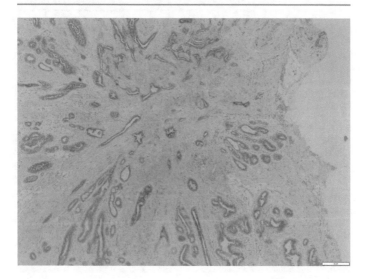

Fig. 4.11 Radial scar with the fibro-elastotic centre containing small distorted ducts that can be confused with a tubular carcinoma

glands in the middle of the fibro-elastotic scar can be easily confused with a small focus of a tubular carcinoma (Fig. 4.11) or a low grade ductal carcinoma (Fig. 4.12). Positive staining for myoepithelial cells, for example p63 (Fig. 4.13), is commonly needed to confirm the benign nature of these distorted glands and exclude the possibility of a tubular carcinoma. Sometimes, particularly in larger complex sclerosing lesions, the central fibro-elastotic scar may not be included in the core biopsy and the diagnosis will rely on the detection of florid epithelial proliferation that proves to be benign by cellular and nuclear morphology (Fig. 4.14a), and by the presence of myoepithelial cells around the proliferating cells (Fig. 4.14b). Atypical ductal hyperplasia, flat epithelial atypia and in situ lobular neoplasia may be present, and if so they should be mentioned in the report and in the conclusion as management will be different.

In a published study of 126 radial scars from the Royal Marsden Hospital, most cases with malignant change were larger than 7 mm and occurred in women above the age of 50 years [7]. The incidence of malignancy in that study was relatively high (9.5% in cases

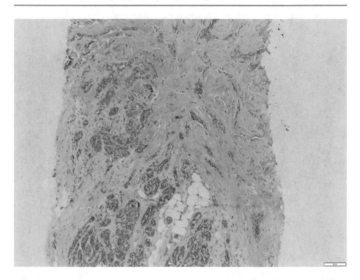

Fig. 4.12 Radial scar with more alarming features suggestive of malignancy

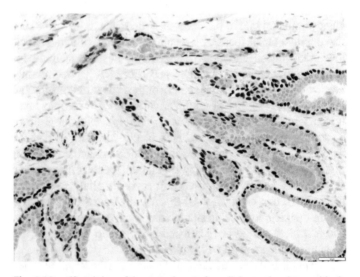

Fig. 4.13 p63 staining of the central part of a radial scar showing positively stained myoepithelial cells around the distorted and proliferative ducts

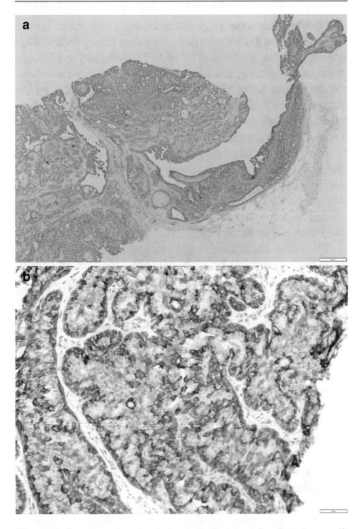

Fig. 4.14 Complex sclerosing lesion including part of an intraduct papilloma: (**a**) H&E; (**b**) CK5 staining showing a mosaic pattern of positive (basal/myoepithelial) and negative (Luminal) cells

derived from the routine surgical service, and 19% in referral cases). The carcinomas described in that series were mostly DCIS, of low and high nuclear grade, with a few LCIS cases, and four invasive carcinomas including two tubular and two grade 2 invasive ductal [7]. In another series of 17 radial scars with neoplasia from The Armed Forces Institute of Pathology, eight had in situ lobular neoplasia, three intermediate grade DCIS and six had invasive carcinoma including one tubular and five grade 1 invasive ductal [8].

Five cases of metaplastic carcinoma [9] and five cases of spindle cell lesions, including three cases of fibromatosis and two of fibrosarcoma [10], have also been described developing in radial scars and complex sclerosing lesions. Nine patients varied in age between 49 and 79 years, the tenth patient was 24 year old who developed fibromatosis. The lesion varied in sizes between 7 and 25 mm.

There seems to be a higher risk (×1.8) of developing carcinoma in patients with benign biopsies containing radial scars than those without scars [11], but a direct link between radial scars and invasive carcinoma has not been definitely established.

In a recent meta-analysis of 3163 reported cases of radial scars/ complex sclerosing lesions diagnosed on core or vacuum biopsy, 7% were upgraded to DCIS or invasive carcinoma on excision [12]. The rate of upgrading varied according to the presence or absence of atypia and according to whether the diagnosis was made by a 14G core biopsy or by vacuum assisted biopsy. For core biopsies, the upgrade was 5% for cases with no atypia and 29% in cases with atypia. For Vacuum biopsies the corresponding rates were 1 and 18%. The current recommendation is to manage cases of radial scars and complex sclerosing lesions with no atypia with vacuum excision [1]. If ADH, FEA or ILN are present, the protocol for these lesions is followed (see above).

Intraduct Papillomas

Benign intraduct papillomas are discrete intraductal polypoid lesions with arborizing fibro-vascular stroma covered by two layers of cells: a myoepithelial layer and a columnar or cuboidal epithelial layer [13] (Fig. 4.15a, b). They are usually divided

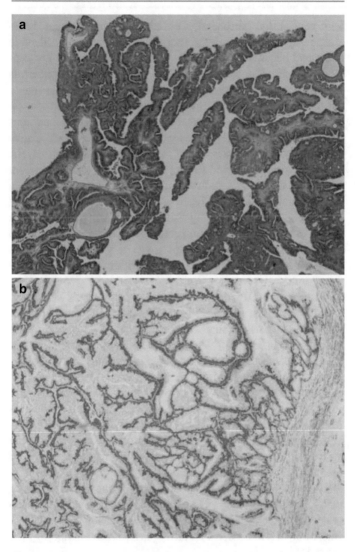

Fig. 4.15 Benign intraduct papilloma: (**a**) H&E; (**b**) CK5 staining showing a mosaic pattern of positive and negative cells

into central and peripheral. Central, usually subareolar, intraduct papillomas are mostly single but can reach considerable sizes and become symptomatic. Peripheral papillomas are generally smaller, but may be multiple and recurrent. A patient is usually considered to have multiple papillomas if she has five or more. Excessive epithelial proliferation i.e. hyperplasia may be present. The latter is defined as the presence of more than four layers of epithelial cells covering the papillary fronds and can be of the regular or atypical type [14]. In regular hyperplasia, the cells are not uniform and show a mixed mosaic staining pattern with CK5 (Fig. 4.16). In atypical hyperplasia, the proliferating cells are uniform (Fig. 4.17a, b) and are CK5 negative. Rounded spaces may be present giving rise to a cribriform pattern, but the affected area is less than 3 mm across [14]. If more than that, the lesion is considered DCIS and given a score of B5a [14]. Atypical hyperplasia may be present within or adjacent to the papilloma.

In a review of 9108 benign breast cases, papillomas were found in 480 (5%). Most of these (372; 78%) were single with no atypia, while 54 (11%) were single with atypia, 41 (8%) were multiple without atypia and 13 (2%) were multiple with atypia [13]. The relative risk of breast cancer development in this large series was **2** for patients with single papillomas and no atypia (similar to proliferative breast disease without atypia), **3** for patients with multiple papillomas and no atypia, **5** for patients with single papillomas with atypia and **7** for patients with multiple papillomas with atypia [13]. In another study, the presence of cellular atypia within, or outside, the papilloma is associated with a fourfold increased risk of carcinoma. When the latter develops it usually arises in the same breast and possibly nearer the site of the previously excised papilloma [14, 15]. Papillomas may show wide areas of sclerosis, particularly in post-menopausal women. Microcalcification, infarction and squamous metaplasia my also occur [16].

Small intraduct papillomas that appear completely excised in a core biopsy is usually given a B2 sore with no further treatment needed (Fig. 4.18) Intraduct papilloma with no atypia, can be excised with a vacuum biopsy. Large intraduct papillomas and papillomas with atypia require surgical excision [1].

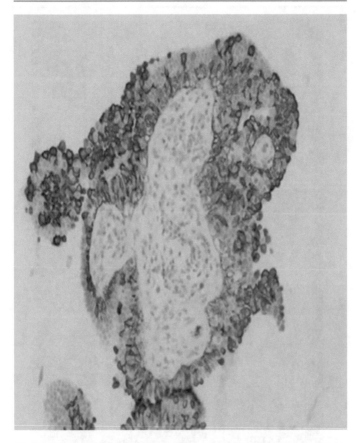

Fig. 4.16 CK5 staining of a frond of a benign intraduct papilloma with epithelial hyperplasia. Note the presence of the mosaic pattern of staining

There seems to be a separate entity that used to be called juvenile papillomatosis which is characterised by the presence of numerous closely packed small intraduct papillomas, producing a worrying palpable lump that can be clinically confused with carcinoma (Fig. 4.19). The cellular morphology (Fig. 4.20a) and positive immunohistochemistry for myoepithelial/basal cell markers (Fig. 4.20b) would help in confirming the benign nature of the disease. Occasionally however foci of DCIS may be seen dispersed in the lesion (Figs. 4.21a–c and 4.22a, b); hence the whole lesion has

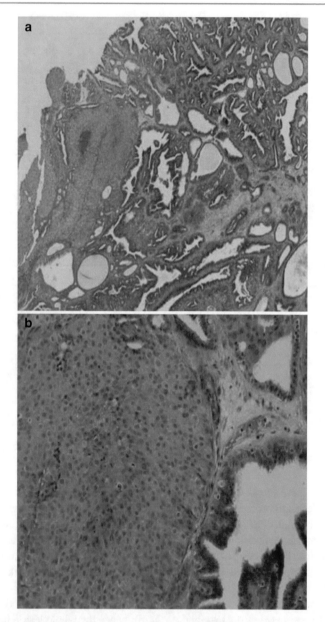

Fig. 4.17 (**a**) Intraduct papilloma with an area of atypical hyperplasia, on the left hand side, with a solid area of larger more uniform cells. (**b**) High power of the atypical area

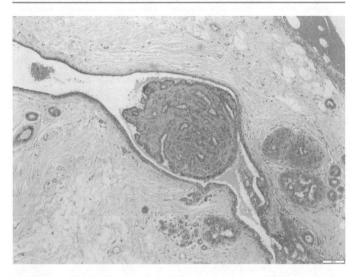

Fig. 4.18 A completely excised small benign intraduct papilloma. This if on its own would be scored as B2

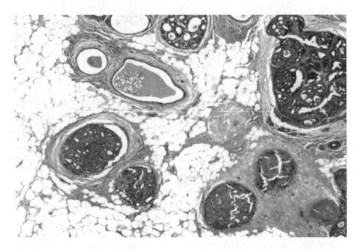

Fig. 4.19 'Juvenile' papillomatosis. Note the absence of fibrous cores between the proliferating intraductal epithelial cells

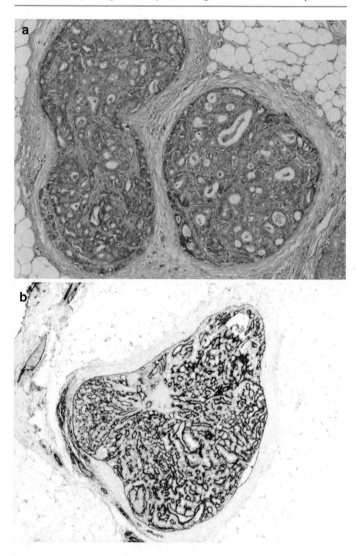

Fig. 4.20 'Juvenile' papillomatosis, high power view of the same lesion seen in Fig. 4.19: (**a**) H&E; (**b**) CD10 immunostaining, a basal/myoepithelial marker, showing a mosaic pattern of staining

to be thoroughly examined and several sections may have to be stained for CK5 to exclude or confirm the presence of DCIS which would change the management. The lesion was first described by Rosen in 1980 [17] who wrote again about the subject in 1982 [18], 1883 [19] and 1990 [20]. Rosen defined the lesion as papillary hyperplasia involving multiple ducts involving large area of the breast with most proliferations have no fibrous stroma (in contrast to intraduct papillomas). Cysts are usually present giving rise to a 'Swiss cheese' appearance of the gross specimen. The age incidence is 30s and 40s [21]. The lesions can be bilateral. Ten per cent of 41 patients reported by Rosen developed breast carcinoma, all had recurrent and bilateral involvement [20]. It must be said here that the term juvenile papillomatosis is not accepted by all authors who consider the disease as an example of peripheral multiple intraduct papillomas. However, whatever name is used the disease exists and has specific morphology and associations as illustrated by Rosen and by our cases presented here (Figs. 4.21 and 4.22).

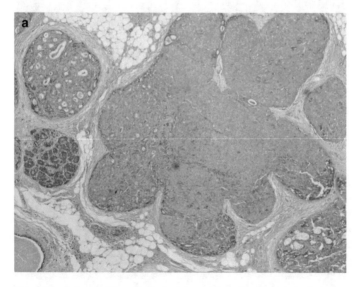

Fig. 4.21 A focus of low grade ductal carcinoma in situ seen in the same case depicted in Figs. 4.19 and 4.20. (**a**) H&E, low power; (**b**) H&E high power, (**c**) CD10 staining showing negative staining of the malignant area

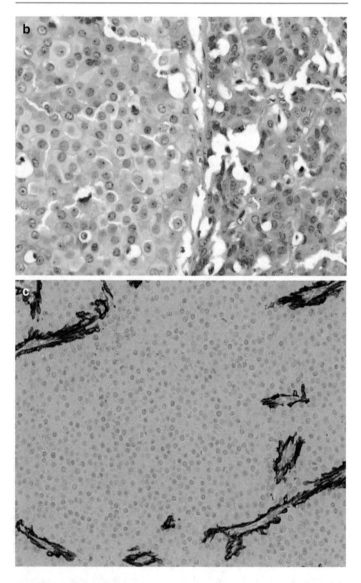

Fig. 4.21 (continued)

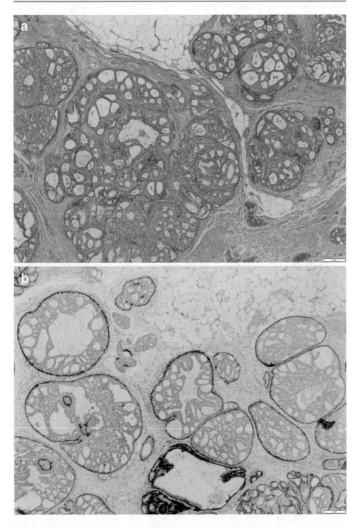

Fig. 4.22 A different case of 'Juvenile' papillomatosis including foci of low grade cribriform DCIS. (**a**) H&E (**b**) CK5 staining demonstrating the lack of its expression in the malignant cells

Cellular Fibro-Epithelial Lesions

These are lesions that have features similar to those seen in fibro-adenomas, but with the added element of mild to moderate stromal hypercellularity [22] (Fig. 4.23). The idea of using this term is to indicate that the possibility of phyllodes tumour cannot be excluded. Several criteria have been described trying to distinguish phyllodes tumours from cellular fibroadenomas, but none of these criteria is perfect and distinguishing the two lesions stays difficult, hence the use of the term cellular fibroepithelial lesion with a B score of 3 indicating that further clinical action is needed, which should be surgical excision with a safety margin [1]. Histological features in core biopsies that have been suggested to be more in favour of phyllodes tumour include fragmentation of the cores, stromal hypercellularity and overgrowth, condensation of stroma around epithelial elements, stromal nuclear pleomorphism and more than 3 mitotic figure/10 HPF [23].

It has to be mentioned here that a degree of stromal hypercellularity and mitotic activity is not uncommon in juvenile fibroade-

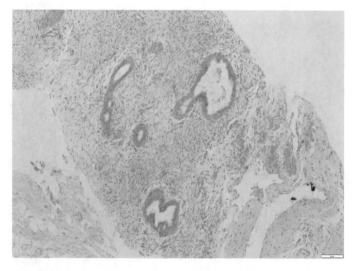

Fig. 4.23 Cellular fibro-epithelial lesion with moderately hypercellular stroma

nomas developing in adolescents and young women [22], but these are usually scored as B2 as long as there are no other alarming features like excessive mitosis (more than 2/10 HPF) or extensive stromal cellularity and nuclear atypia.

Spindle Cell Lesions

All spindle cell lesions of the breast are given a score of B3 at least. B5 is given if there is a high probability of malignancy. The first step in dealing with a breast spindle cell lesion in a core biopsy is to do cytokeratin immunostains to exclude the possibility of a spindle cell carcinoma. There is no single cytokeratin stain that can positively stain all epithelial lesions of the breast, hence at least two stains have to be tried. We usually use MNF116 and AE1/AE3 which would detect most spindle cell carcinomas. If these two are negative and there is a high possibility of carcinoma, more stains are used including CK5, 18, 19 and p63. The latter is thought to be positive in many metaplastic breast carcinomas including spindle cell ones.

Once the possibility of spindle cell carcinoma has been excluded, the next step is to decide whether the lesion is benign or malignant. H&E stained sections are usually enough for this step. The presence of high cellularity, marked nuclear pleomorphism, abundant mitosis or the presence of areas of necrosis all point to a malignant soft tissue tumour. The presence of dispersed benign glandular elements would be in favour of a malignant phyllodes tumour. Even in the absence of such glandular elements, a malignant phyllodes would still be the strongest possibility. Once malignancy is excluded the lesion will be scored as B3 with a differential diagnosis including fibromatosis and other rare breast lesions like myofibroblastoma, nodular fasciitis, solitary fibrous tumour. Positive staining for ER and Androgen receptors are in favour of myofibroblastoma, as well as the occasional presence of fat cells (Fig. 4.24). Positive staining for CD34 favours phyllodes tumour, while nuclear beta-catenin is more common in fibromatosis. S100 is positive in neurofibromas (Fig. 4.25) and Schwannomas. In the absence of any distinguishing features, a differential diagnosis and a score of B3 is given with

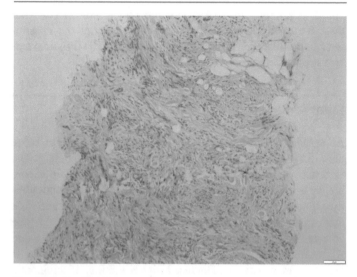

Fig. 4.24 Myofibroblastoma. Note the presence of fat cells and short bundles of spindle shaped cells that were positive for desmin and ER

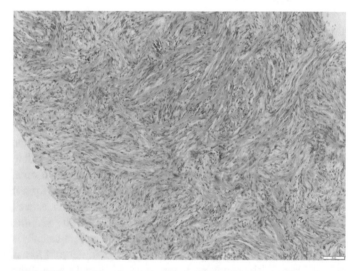

Fig. 4.25 Neurofibroma. Highly cellular spindle cell lesion that was positive for S100

recommendation of surgical excision [1]. The only lesion that is currently thought better left alone is fibromatosis. The radiological appearance might help as it usually has an infiltrative pattern and microscopically the spindle cells are bland, arranged in waves (Fig. 4.26a) that surround rather than infiltrate the glandular elements of the breast (Fig. 4.26b). The lesions show strong nuclear

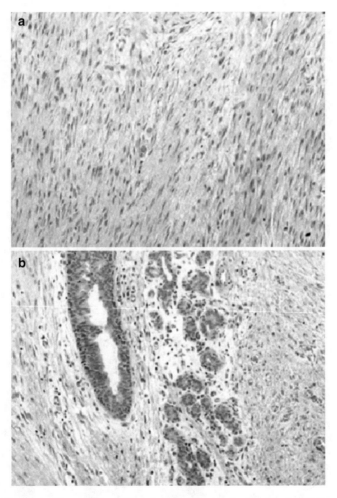

Fig. 4.26 Fibromatosis. (**a**) Bundles of bland spindle shaped cells, (**b**) that insinuates between the preserved glandular structures

beta catenin staining. Leiomyoma is another benign spindle cell lesion that can be positively diagnosed as it express desmin and smooth muscle actin. Rare solitary fibrous tumours have been seen in the breast (Fig. 4.27a). Characteristically the lesions are positive for STAT6 and can be positive for SMA, beta catenin and Bcl2 (Fig. 4.27b).

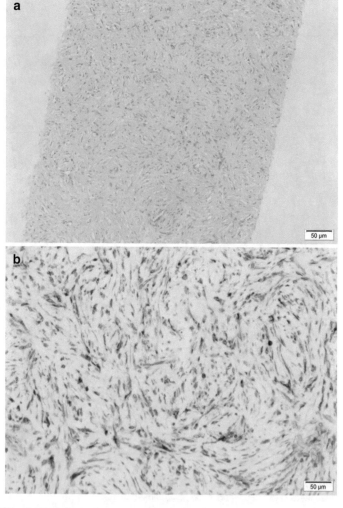

Fig. 4.27 Solitary fibrous tumour. (**a**) H&E (**b**) positive staining with Bcl 2

Mucocele Like Lesions

This is a spectrum of lesions characterised by the presence of cysts containing acidic mucin which may rupture causing extravasation of the mucin into the adjacent breast stroma (Fig. 4.28a). The mucin stains blue with alcian blue/PAS stain (Fig. 4.28b). The lesions are usually detected during mammographic screening because of the presence of abundant fine microcalcification within

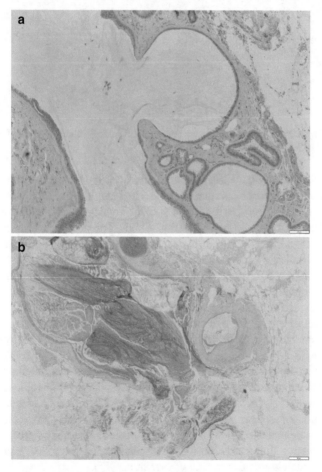

Fig. 4.28 Mucocele-like lesion. (**a**) H&E; (**b**) Alcian blue/PAS staining demonstrating the presence of alcian blue positive acidic mucin

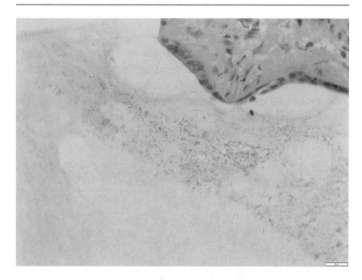

Fig. 4.29 Mucocele-like lesion demonstrating abundant fine microcalcification floating in the mucin

the mucin (Fig. 4.29). The epithelial cyst lining may be simple flat, cuboidal or columnar (Fig. 4.30a), atypical flat (Fig. 4.30b) atypical hyperplastic (Fig. 4.30c) or frankly in situ malignant leading to mucinous DCIS (Fig. 4.30d). The lining epithelium is always ER strongly positive and CK5 negative. Detached epithelial cells may be sometimes found within intracystic or extracystic mucin, which makes them difficult to distinguish from invasive mucinous carcinoma. The configuration of the lesion and the absence of fibrous stroma in the mucous lakes help to differentiate them from invasive carcinomas. In a series of 39 cases seen on core biopsies, 33% were associated with ADH and 10% with DCIS [24]. All mucocele-like lesions are WT1 positive [25] (Fig. 4.31) which links them to invasive mucinous carcinomas, as around 60% of mucinous carcinomas are WT1 positive [26]. This supports the previously suggested concept that there is a continuum of lesions representing a specific pathway progressing through mucin filled ducts, to mucocele-like lesions with progressing lining from normal to atypical, to mucinous DCIS and ultimately invasive mucinous carcinoma [27].

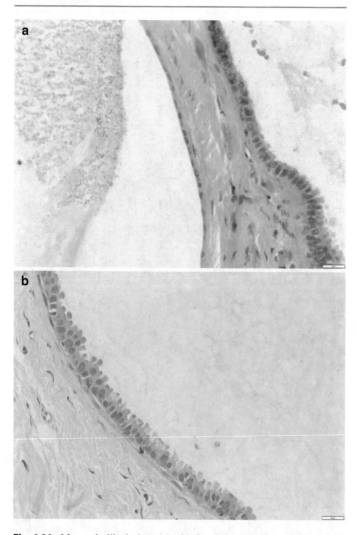

Fig. 4.30 Mucocele-like lesion: (**a**) with flat (left) and columnar cell (right) lining; (**b**) flat epithelial atypia type lining; (**c**) lining showing features of atypical ductal hyperplasia; (**d**) lining showing features of intermediate grade DCIS

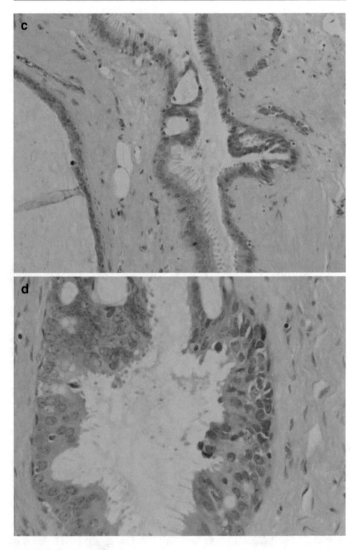

Fig. 4.30 (continued)

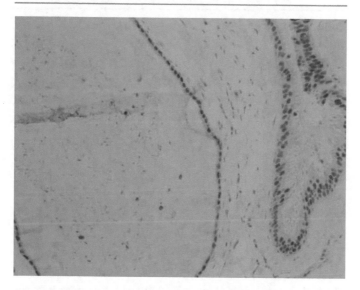

Fig. 4.31 Mucocele-like lesion. Positive staining for WT1

Of 57 cases diagnosed by core biopsy at Charing Cross Hospital, London, 31 (54%) had no atypia, 23 showed atypia and 3 showed changes amounting to DCIS. Of 35 non-malignant cases surgically excised, none of the 18 cases with no atypia showed atypia or malignancy on excision, while 4 (25%) out of 16 cases with atypia in the core showed low grade DCIS on excision. These findings are similar to other reported in the literature [28] and suggest that in the absence of atypia, vacuum excision would be an adequate treatment and that surgical excision is needed if there is atypia in the core.

The differential diagnosis of mucocele like lesions include: cysts of fibrocystic change: no mucin; duct ectasia: no mucin but peri-ductal fibrosis and inflammation; Galactocele: no mucin but history of pregnancy or lactation and the usual presence of lactational change; cystic pseudo-lactational hyperplasia: no acidic mucin and there are lactational changes in lining cells and sometimes psammoma-like microcalcification in the lumen (Fig. 4.32); Cystic hyersecretory hyperplasia and DCIS: no mucin, but there may be acidophilic secretion.

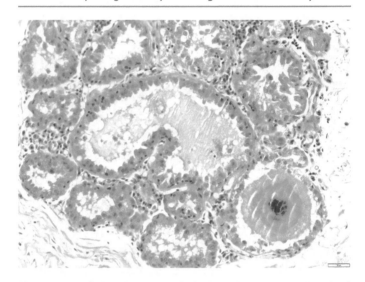

Fig. 4.32 Pseudo-lactational hyperplasia. The epithelium shows lactational change with eosinophilic secretion and psammoma-like microcalcification in the lumen

Microglandular Adenosis

This is a benign proliferative glandular lesion that can mimic tubular carcinoma clinically and histologically. The condition may be rarely present on its own as a breast mass, but is more commonly seen as a part of a benign fibrocystic change lesion or in association with a variety of carcinomas which will be discussed later. Age incidence is 28–82 years, with most patients being 45–55. Characteristically, the lesion consists of haphazardly scattered small uniform rounded glands lined by a single layer of cuboidal epithelium, and having well-defined lumina containing a drop of eosinophilic secretion that is PAS positive (Fig. 4.33a). The stroma is bland, with no evidence of desmoplasia. The glands are 'naked' with no surrounding myoepithelium but are ER negative and S100 strongly positive (Fig. 4.33b). These latter two features distinguish them from invasive tubular carci-

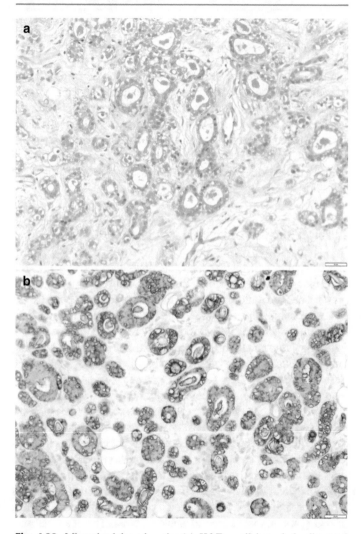

Fig. 4.33 Microglandular adenosis: (**a**) H&E small irregularly dispersed glands some with a drop of eosinophilic secretion in the lumen; (**b**) strong positive staining for S100

noma which is the main differential diagnosis. The lesion is given a B3 score as it is sometimes present adjacent to or associated with carcinoma [29]. Atypical microglandular adenosis has the same basic features of absent myoepithelium, negative ER and positive S100, but in addition atypical features may be present in the form of nuclear atypia, cellular multi-layering and multiple lumina. The atypical form is more commonly seen in association with carcinoma, but if it is seen on its own in a core biopsy A B3 score is still used. As the lesion is probably pre-cancerous or can be associated with carcinoma, surgical excision is probably the most appropriate treatment.

Benign and Atypical Vascular Lesions

Small benign peri-lobular haemangiomas seen incidentally in a core biopsy showing a benign lesion like a fibroadenoma or fibro-cystic change would not change the B score from B2 to B3. On the other hand, it is usually advised that larger benign lesions presenting as radiological distortions are to be given a score of B3 with a recommendation for surgical excisions, to avoid bleeding and to confirm the absence of malignancy. Examples of such lesions include capillary (Fig. 4.34a, b) and cavernous (Fig. 4.35) hamangiomas and angio-lipomas (Fig. 4.36).

Atypical vascular lesions are sometimes seen in punch biopsies of the breast skin in patients with past history of carcinoma treated by radiotherapy. These lesions would present clinically as a skin discolouration of an area that has been previously irradiated. The important thing is to exclude angiosarcoma, which can develop in a similar situation. The punch biopsy will show variable numbers of dilated thin-walled vascular channels lined by endothelial cells showing a minimal degree of nuclear atypia. The channels may dissect between collagen bundles, but there is no papillary or solid proliferation of the lining atypical endothelial cells (Fig. 4.37a–c). Immunohistochemistry for C-MYC is negative in contrast to post-irradiation angiosarcoma where the neoplastic endothelial cells show strong nuclear expression of C-MYC [30]. Rarely, dilatation

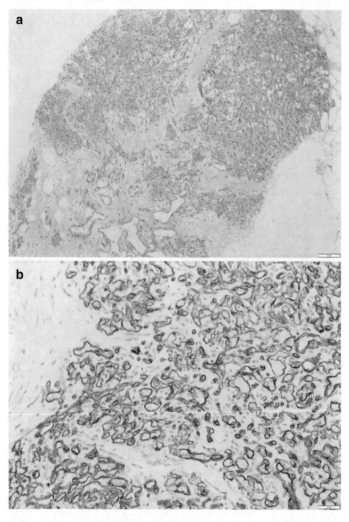

Fig. 4.34 Lobulated capillary haemangioma. (**a**) H&E; (**b**) Positive staining of the endothelial cells lining the capillaries with CD34

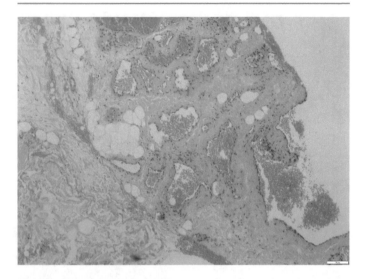

Fig. 4.35 Cavernous haemangioma

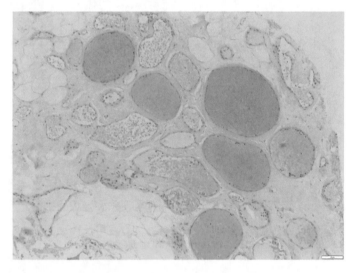

Fig. 4.36 Angiolipoma: a mixture of fat and thin-walled blood vessels

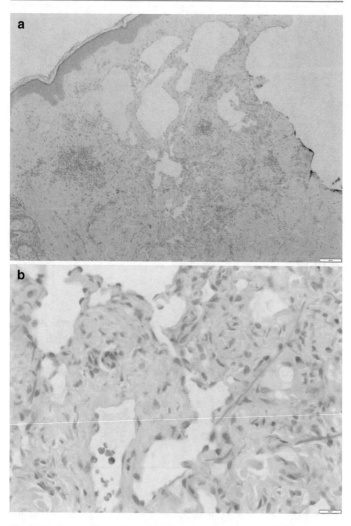

Fig. 4.37 Atypical vascular lesion, skin punch biopsy: (**a**) H&E Low power view to show dissection of vascular spaces between collagen fibres; (**b**) H&E high power view showing endothelial cells with slightly enlarged darkly stained endothelial cells; (**c**) CD31 staining showing the positively stained interconnected blood vessels

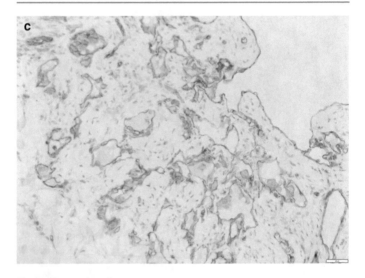

Fig. 4.37 (continued)

of superficial lymphatics can occur after radiotherapy, resulting in clinically identifiable lesions which can amount to a small, sometimes multiple, lymphangiomas (Fig. 4.38a, b). These atypical vascular lesions are also given a score of B3 with recommendation of surgical excision for the reasons given above and in particular to exclude the possibility of angiosarcoma. Small published studies however failed to show upgrading of none atypical and atypical vascular lesions on excision [31].

Granular Cell Tumour

An uncommon lesion, usually solitary, that can occur in the breasts of female and male patients of any age. Size can vary from under 1 cm up to 6 cm. Radiologically, the lesions Usually appear circumscribed, but may have infiltrative borders. The core biopsy shows closely packed relatively large sheets and nests of large polygonal cells with faintly stained granular cytoplasm and small rounded nuclei (Fig. 4.39a). The lesion in the core may appear infiltrative with irregular margin, if the margin was included in the

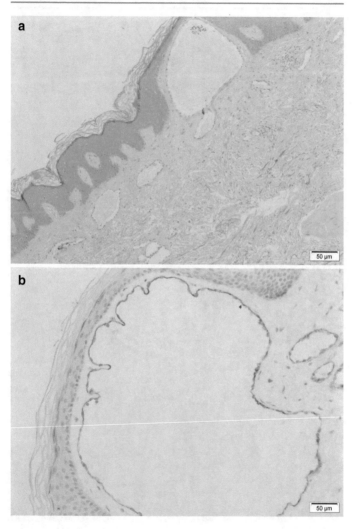

Fig. 4.38 Dilated lymphatic vessels in a skin punch biopsy from a patient with past history of breast cancer treated with radiotherapy: (**a**) H&E; (**b**) positive staining of the lymphatics with D2-40

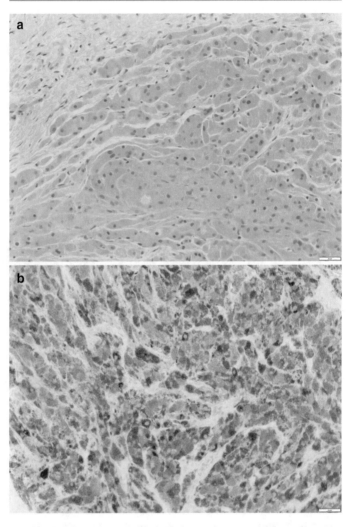

Fig. 4.39 Granular cell tumour (**a**) H&E; (**b**) strong positive staining with S100

biopsy, which may raise the possibility of carcinoma. But the nuclei are small and show no evidence of atypia. Mitosis and nuclear pleomorphism are unusual. Small nerve bundles may be seen within the lesion or near-by. More important, the cells are ER negative and S100 strongly positive (Fig. 4.39b). The cytoplasmic granules are PAS positive, diastase resistant. Most lesions are benign, but rare malignant granular cell tumours have been described in various organs including the breast [32].

Collagenous Spherulosis

This is an extremely uncommon lesion, usually seen in association with other diseases which could be benign like fibrocystic change or neoplastic particularly in situ lobular neoplasia. The lesion has a cribriform pattern (Fig. 4.40a), hence it has to be differentiated from other malignant cribriform lesions of the breast particularly cribriform DCIS and adenoid cystic carcinoma.

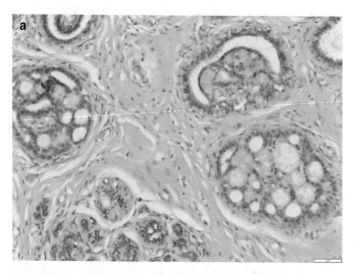

Fig. 4.40 Collagenous spheriolosis: (**a**) H&E; (**b**) Laminin staining the basement membrane as well as surrounding the cribriform cavities

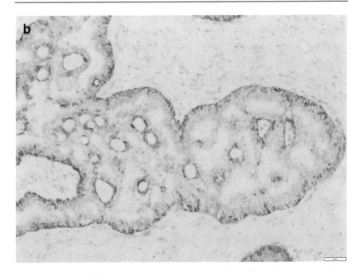

Fig. 4.40 (continued)

In contrast to Cribriform DCIS, Collagenous spheriolosis is usually ER negative. The cavities in collagenous spheriolosis contain basement membrane material which is positive for Laminin (Fig. 4.40b) and Collagen 4, which are absent in the cavities of cribriform and adenoid cystic carcinomas.

Epithelial Myoepithelial Benign Lesions

Rarely a core biopsy might show an epithelial lesion associated with marked proliferation of myoepithelial cells (Fig. 4.41a–c). Both elements appear benign with no evidence of nuclear atypia or obvious mitotic activity. The differential diagnosis would include benign adenomyoepithelioma and pleomorphic adenoma of the breast. These lesions should be given a score of B3 with recommendation of surgical excision as the natural history of these lesions is not clear. Some adenomyoepitheliomas in particular may harbour malignancy and epithelial myoepithelial carcinomas have been seen in the breast.

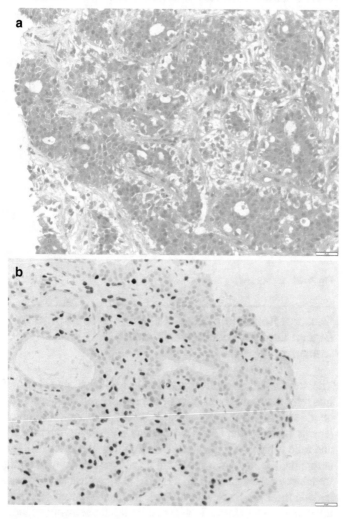

Fig. 4.41 Epithelial myoepithelial lesion: (**a**) H&E showing darkly stained luminal epithelium and pale stained myoepithelial cells; (**b**) p63 positive staining of myoepithelial cells; (**c**) ER mosaic staining pattern: positive luminal and negative myoepithelial cells

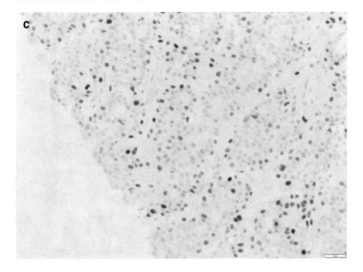

Fig. 4.41 (continued)

General Remark: Risk of Malignancy in Benign Breast Lesions Discovered During Mammography

The non-mass forming benign breast lesions have been classified into three main categories: non-proliferative, Proliferative without atypia and atypical hyperplasia [33, 34]. The non-proliferative lesions include simple cysts, apocrine metaplasia, duct ectasia and mild usual type hyperplasia. The Proliferative lesions with no atypia include moderate and florid usual type ductal hyperplasia, intraduct papilloma and radial scars. The atypical hyperplasias include those involving ducts (atypical ductal hyperplasia), those involving lobules (In situ lobular neoplasia), those involving intra-duct papillomas (Intraduct papillomas with atypia) and atypical apocrine adenosis. The risk of developing cancer has been estimated to be 1.17 in non-proliferative lesions, 1.76 in proliferative lesions with no atypia and 3.93 in atypical hyperplasia [33, 34]. Most of these lesions are detected by mammographic screening, although occasionally the patient may present with a palpable lump or nipple discharge. Other uncommon benign breast lesions with undetermined risk factor that are usually detected by mammography include sclerosing adenosis, microglandular adenosis and mucocele-like lesions.

Mass producing benign breast lesions include fibroadenoma, tubular adenoma, lactating adenoma, benign phyllodes tumour, myofibroblastoma, nodular fasciitis, fibromatosis and granular cell tumour. These lesions are not known to be associated with an increased risk of developing carcinoma.

References

1. Rageth CJ, O'Flynn EAM, Pinker K, et al. Second international consensus conference on lesions of uncertain malignant potential in the breast (B3 lesions). Breast Cancer Res Treat. 2019;174:279–96.
2. Ouldamer L, Poisson E, Arbion F, et al. All pure flat atypical atypia lesions of the breast diagnosed using percutaneous vacuum-assisted breast biopsy do not need surgical excision. Breast. 2018;40:4–9.
3. Dawn Forester N, Lowes S, Mitchell E, Twiddy M. High risk (B3) breast lesions: what is the incidence of malignancy for individual lesion subtypes? A systematic review and meta-analysis. Eur J Surg Oncol. 2019;45:519–27.
4. Shousha S. In situ lobular neoplasia of the breast with marked myoepithelial proliferation. Histopathology. 2011;58:1081–5.
5. Shousha S, Forbes G, Hopkins I, Wright G. CD10 positive myoepithelial cells are usually prominent around in situ lobular neoplasia of the breast and much less prominent or absent in DCIS. J Clin Pathol. 2016;69(7):702–5.
6. Nakhlis F, Harrison BT, Giess CS, et al. Evaluating the rate of upgrade to invasive breast cancer and/or ductal carcinoma in situ following a core biopsy diagnosis of *non-classic* lobular carcinoma in situ. Ann Surg Oncol. 2019;26:55–61.
7. Sloane JP, Mayers MM. Carcinoma and atypical hyperplasia in radial scars and complex sclerosing lesions: importance of lesion size and patient age. Histopathology. 1993;23:225–31.
8. Alvarado-Cabrero I, Tavassoli FA. Neoplastic and malignant lesions involving or arising in a radial scar: a clinicopathologic analysis of 17 cases. Breast J. 2000;6:96–102.
9. Denley H, Pinder SE, Tan PH, Sim CS, Brown R, Barker T, Gearty J, Elston CW, Ellis IO. Metaplastic carcinoma of the breast arising within complex sclerosing lesion: a report of five cases. Histopathology. 2000;36:203–9.

10. Gobbi H, Simpson JF, Jensen RA, Olson SJ, Page DL. Metaplastic spindle cell breast tumors arising within papillomas, complex sclerosing lesions, and nipple adenomas. Mod Pathol. 2003;16:893–901.

11. Jacobs TW, Byrne C, Colditz G, Connolly JL, Schnitt SJ. Radial scars in benign breast biopsy specimens and the risk of breast cancer. N Engl J Med. 1999;340:430–6.

12. Farshid G, Buckley E. Meta-analysis of upgrade rates in 3163 radial scars excised after needle biopsy diagnosis. Breast Cancer Res Treat. 2019;174:165–77.

13. Lewis JT, Hartmann LC, Vierkant RA, Maloney SD, Pankratz S, Allers TM, Frost MH, Visscher DW. An analysis of breast cancer risk in women with single, multiple, and atypical papilloma. Am J Surg Pathol. 2006;30:665–72.

14. Page DL, Salhany KE, Jensen RA, Dupont WD. Subsequent breast carcinoma risk after biopsy with atypia in a breast papilloma. Cancer. 1996;78:258–66.

15. Raju U, Vertes D. Breast papillomas with atypical ductal hyperplasia: a clinico-pathological study. Hum Pathol. 1996;27:1231–8.

16. Flint A, Oberman HA. Infarction and squamous metaplasia in intraductal papilloma: a benign breast lesion that may simulate carcinoma. Hum Pathol. 1984;15:764–7.

17. Rosen PP, et al. Juvenile papillomatosis (Swiss cheese disease) of the breast. In: Fenoglio CD, Wolff M, editors. Progress in surgical pathology, vol. 1. New York: Masson Publishing; 1980. p. 245–54.

18. Rosen PP, et al. Juvenile papillomatosis of the breast and family history of breast carcinoma. Cancer. 1982;49:2591–5.

19. Rosen PP, et al. Juvenile papillomatosis and breast carcinoma. Cancer. 1985;55:1345–52.

20. Rosen PP, Kimmel M. Juvenile papillomatosis of the breast. A follow up study of 41 patients having biopsies before 1979. Am J Clin Pathol. 1990;93:599–603.

21. Bazzocchi F, et al. Juvenile papillomatosis (epitheliosis) of the breast. A clinical and pathologic study of 13 cases. Am J Clin Pathol. 1986;86:745–8.

22. Krings G, Bean GR, Chen Y-Y. Fibroepithelial lesions: the WHO spectrum. Semin Diagn Pathol. 2017;34:438–52.

23. Lee AHS, Hodi Z, Ellis IO, Elston CW. Histological features useful in the distinction of phyllodes tumour and fibroadenoma on needle core biopsy of the breast. Histopathology. 2007;51:336–44.

24. Khodeza SM, Begum N, Jara-Lazaro AR, Thike AA, Tse GM-K, Wong JS-L, Ho JT-S, Tan PH. Mucin extravasation in breast core biopsies—clinical significance and outcome correlation. Histopathology. 2009;55:609–17.

25. Shousha S, Ali N. WT1 is expressed in a continuum of breast lesions extending from simple mucinous cysts to mucocele-like lesions, muci-

nous DCIS and invasive mucinous carcinoma. Virchows Arch. 2015;467(Suppl 1):S51.

26. Damfeh AB, Carley AL, Striobel JM, et al. WT1 immunoreactivity in breast carcinoma: selective expression in pure and mixed mucinous subtypes. Mod Pathol. 2008;21:1217–23.

27. Weaver MG, Abdul-karim FW, Al-Kaisi N. Mucinous lesions of the breast: a pathological continuum. Pathol Res Pract. 1993;189:873–6.

28. Zhang G, Ataya D, Lebda P, Calhoun BC. Mucocele-like lesions diagnosed on breast core biopsy: risk of upgrade and subsequent carcinoma. Breast J. 2018;24:314–8.

29. Khalifeh IM, Albarracin C, Diaz LK, Symmans FW, Edgerton ME, Hwang RF, Sneige N. Clinical, histopathologic, and immunohistochemical features of microglandular adenosis and transition into in situ and invasive carcinoma. Am J Surg Pathol. 2008;32:544–52.

30. Ronen S, Ivan D, Torres-Cabala CA, et al. Post-radiation vascular lesions of the breast. J Cutan Pathol. 2019;46:52–8.

31. Sebastiano C, Gennaro L, Brogi E, et al. Benign vascular lesions of the breast diagnosed by core needle biopsy do not require excision. Histopathology. 2017;71:795–804.

32. Khansur T, Balducci L, Tavassoli M. Granular cell tumor. Clinical spectrum of the benign and malignant entity. Cancer. 1987;60:220–2.

33. Pearlman MD, Griffin JI. Benign breast disease. Obstet Gynecol. 2010;116:747–58.

34. Dyrstad SW, Yan Y, Fowler AM, Colditz GA. Breast cancer risk associated with benign breast disease: systematic review and meta-analysis. Breast Cancer Res Treat. 2015;149:569–75.

Reporting Core Biopsies: Lesions That Are Highly Suspicious of Malignancy (B4) or Definitely Malignant (B5)

5

B4 Lesions

This is probably the least used B score for core biopsies. It is only used in the rare situations where there is a strong clinical and radiological evidence of malignancy, but the quality of the biopsy or the number of cells available for assessment are not enough to make a diagnosis. A repeat biopsy is usually needed to establish the diagnosis. Examples of that include biopsies composed mostly of blood with a scanty few atypical cells present, and biopsies suffering from inappropriate fixation or processing.

B5 Lesions

These are core biopsies showing a malignant process which may be in situ, i.e. non-invasive (B5a) or invasive (B5b). All in situ lesions are carcinomas of epithelial origin. Most invasive breast tumours are also carcinomas, but sarcomas and lymphomas are occasionally seen. A diagnosis of malignancy is usually a straightforward process, but sometimes deeper sections or immunohistochemistry may be needed for confirmation or to decide whether the disease is invasive or non-invasive. In these situations a report should not be issued until the results of any extra tests requested became available and a firm diagnosis is given. Giving the patient a diagnosis or even a preliminary

© Springer Nature Switzerland AG 2020
S. Shousha, *Breast Pathology in Clinical Practice*, In Clinical Practice, https://doi.org/10.1007/978-3-030-42386-5_5

diagnosis that later on proves to be wrong is not acceptable as it can lead to un-necessary psychological trauma.

B5a (Non-invasive Lesions)

In Situ Carcinoma

In situ carcinoma is characterised by the presence of an intact basement membrane separating the proliferating malignant cells from the adjacent stroma. It can arise within ducts (ductal carcinoma in situ or DCIS), within the acini of the breast lobules (lobular carcinoma in situ or LCIS), within the epithelium covering the nipple (Paget's disease of the nipple), or within the lining of a cyst (intracystic papillary carcinoma). Myoepithelial cells are usually present, except in Paget's disease, between the basement membrane and the malignant cells. Sometimes, however, they may be attenuated and difficult to demonstrate or completely absent, particularly in high grade DCIS [1].

Ductal Carcinoma In Situ (DCIS)

There has been a marked increase in the detection rate of DCIS with the introduction of mammographic screening. Most of the cases discovered are impalpable. They are detected because of the presence of microcalcification. A core biopsy is usually carried out to establish the diagnosis.

Any part of the ductal system, from the sub-areolar lactiferous sinuses down to the terminal ductules, deep within the breast tissue, may be involved. In most cases, only a continuous segment of a given duct with its branches are involved. True multifocal DCIS where separate ducts in different parts of the breast are involved is now considered to be uncommon, and most of the multifocal cases are of the micropapillary type. Involvement of the superficial parts of the ducts near the nipple may be associated with Paget's disease of the nipple. Involvement of the deeper terminal parts of the ducts may be associated with extension of malignant cells into lobular acini, leading to what is known as cancerization of lobules.

Not all DCIS lesions are the same, and there are two ways of classifying them, either according to the nuclear morphology or according to the architectural pattern of the lesion. The two methods are sometimes interconnected. The most important classification, which is thought to be related to prognosis, relies on the nuclear grade of the neoplastic cells and classifies DCIS into low, intermediate and high grade. In low grade DCIS, the cells are uniform, near normal size and the nuclei are 1.5–2.0 times the size of red blood cell or normal duct epithelial nucleus (Fig. 5.1a). In high grade DCIS, the cells are larger and are not polarised toward the basement membrane (Fig. 5.1b). The nuclei are markedly pleomorphic with many being more than 2.5 times the size of RBC or normal duct epithelial nucleus. The nuclei may be vesicular with irregular distribution of chromatin. Prominent nucleoli and frequent mitosis are usually present. Comedo necrosis and microcalcification within the lumen and heavy lymphocytic infiltration around the involved ducts, are commonly seen. The microcalcification can give rise to a characteristic linear appearance in

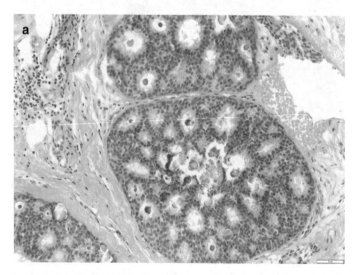

Fig. 5.1 DCIS: (**a**) Low grade, cribriform, with microcalcification, (**b**) High grade, (**c**) intermediate grade

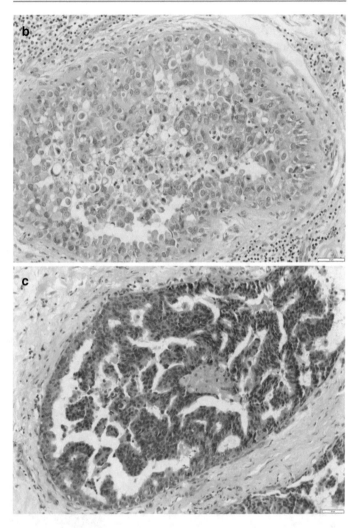

Fig. 5.1 (continued)

x-rays. In intermediate grade DCIS the nuclei show a moderate degree of nuclear pleomorphism which is less than that seen in high grade lesions but lacks the nuclear and cellular monotony of low grade lesions (Fig. 5.1c).

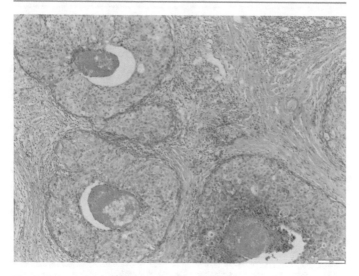

Fig. 5.2 High grade DCIS with central comedo necrosis

DCIS can also be classified according to the histological pattern into comedo, with extensive central necrosis (Fig. 5.2), solid (Fig. 5.1b), cribriform (Fig. 5.1a), micropapillary (Fig. 5.1c), and flat. It is not uncommon to see a mixture of different types and grades in the same lesion; the case should be designated according to the highest grade present. Other less common forms of DCIS include apocrine, mucinous, endocrine and basal types. Apocrine type would be strongly positive for GCDFP-15 (Fig. 5.3). The mucinous type has abundant acidic mucin in the lumen and can be associated with invasive mucinous carcinoma or mucocele-like lesion (Fig. 5.4). The cells in the endocrine type have neuroendocrine granules that would be positive for synaptophysin, chromogranin or CD56. The cells in the basal type are usually homogenously positive for CK5 (Fig. 5.5). Lastly, DCIS can rarely be seen developing in foci of sclerosing adenosis (Fig. 5.6). The basic lobulo-centric architecture of the lesion is preserved but the individual acini forming the lesion are replaced by small solid groups of monomorphic cells that are Ck5 negative and E-cadherin positive.

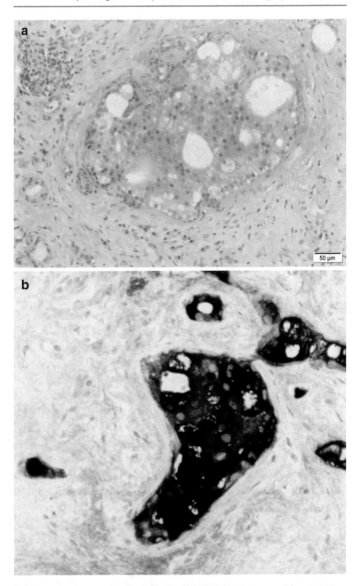

Fig. 5.3 Apocrine DCIS stained with: (**a**) Haematoxylin & Eosin (H&E), (**b**) Gross cystic disease fluid protein (GCDFP)-15, note the intense brown staining

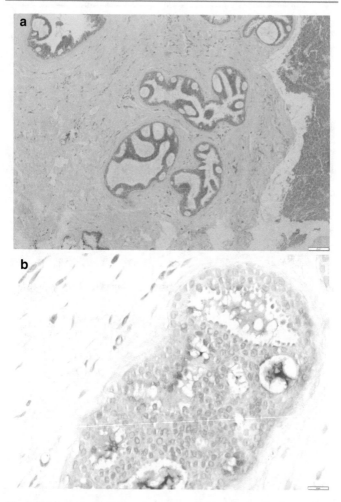

Fig. 5.4 Mucinous DCIS stained with: (**a**) H&E, (**b**) Alcian blue/PAS

The main challenge in diagnosing DCIS in a core biopsy is how to differentiate low grade DCIS from florid usual type and atypical ductal hyperplasia. Immunohistochemistry for cytokeratin 5 is most helpful as discussed in Chap. 3 and Figs. 3.19–3.21. Staining for ER can also provide similar picture. In usual type hyperplasia there is a mosaic pattern of intermingled CK5 posi-

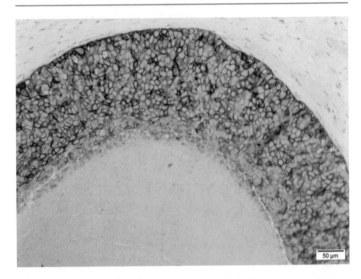

Fig. 5.5 DCIS, basal type, positive strong staining with cytokeratin (CK) 5

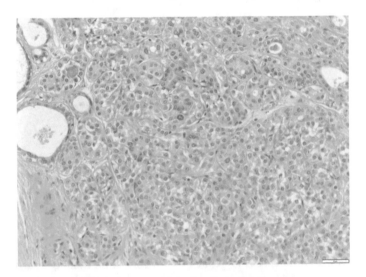

Fig. 5.6 DCIS developing in a focus of sclerosing adenosis

tive and negative cells (Fig. 5.7). In DCIS, the neoplastic cells are usually uniformly negative, except in the rare basal-type mentioned in the paragraph above, although an occasional positive

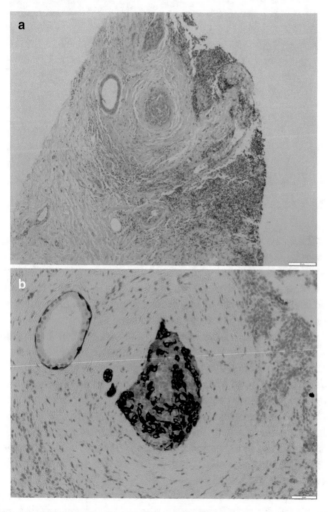

Fig. 5.7 (**a**) A worrying intraductal epithelial proliferation with surrounding fibrosis and lymphocytic infiltration; staininmg for CK 5 (**b**) and Oestrogen receptors (**c**) shows a mosaic appearance of positive and negative cells indicating a benign polymorphic proliferation

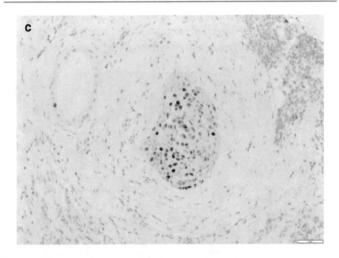

Fig. 5.7   (continued)

cell may be present. In atypical hyperplasia the uniform negative staining is only seen in part of the involved duct or in the whole of a single duct. The principle of considering a single duct involvement as atypical hyperplasia applies only when the neoplastic cells are of low grade. A single duct populated by cells with high or intermediate grade nuclei is considered DCIS.

Immunohistochemical studies have shown that high grade lesions are mostly ER negative and show a high incidence of HER2 and p53 positivity. Low grade lesions are usually ER positive and HER2 and p53 negative. Intermediate grade lesions seem to comprise a mixture of cases with no specific immunoprofile [2]. As some patients now are prescribed Tamoxifen as a prophylactic measure in patients with ER positive lower grades DCIS, assessment of ER is carried out routinely in many centres. Scoring of the result can be carried out on the same basis like in invasive carcinoma (see below).

In reporting core biopsies with DCIS, care has to be taken not to miss an invasive focus, and not to over-diagnose invasion as a result of distortion of the involved duct or Carrey over of tumour cells on the edge of the core biopsy. Extension of DCIS into acini (cancerisation of lobules) can also be mistaken as invasion, but the well-circumscribed appearance of the involved acini should point to the correct diagnosis (Fig. 5.8). If a small focus of invasive carcinoma is seen in a core containing DCIS, the invasive focus should be measured and its size mentioned in the report. The term micro-invasion is not usually used in describing such foci in a core biopsy. The presence of a large focus of calcification within a duct denuded of epithelium or lined by a few atypical cells and surrounded by heavy lymphocytic infiltration should raise the possibility of DCIS, but is not enough to establish the diagnosis and a score of B4 would be more appropriate in that situation particularly if there is radiological suspicion of DCIS. The presence of comedo necrosis is not enough to consider the lesion to be high grade as it can occur, although less common, in lower grades and even sometimes in cases of florid usual type ductal hyperplasia. Also comedo necrosis has to be differentiated from luminal desquamated cells, including macrophages, which can be sometimes seen in the lumen of involved ducts (Fig. 5.1b).

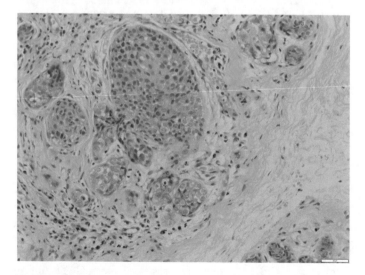

Fig. 5.8 Cancerisation of lobules

Incidence of Metastasis and Death After Diagnosing DCIS

In a study of 108, 196 patients with DCIS, of no specified grade or method of detection, who were followed up for a mean duration of 7.5 years (range 0–23.9), the breast cancer specific mortality was 3.3% and was higher in women diagnosed before the age of 35 years (7.8%) compared with older women (3.2%) [3]. The risk of developing invasive cancer at 20 years was 5.9 in the ipsilateral breast and 6.2% in the contralateral breast. The risk of death increased after the development of an invasive cancer in the same breast. Addition of radiotherapy or mastectomy after removing the primary tumour did not reduce cancer mortality at 10 years [3]. It was concluded that the clinical course of DCIS is similar to that of small invasive cancers [3], which raises the possibility that some of these DCIS cases might have had small invasive cancers that were difficult to detect [4]. In another smaller study of 2123 patients with DCIS, distal metastases developed in 3 patients (0.14%) [4]. The same authors examined 22 further cases that were originally treated in another hospital and found out that the original DCIS showed comedo necrosis in 73.7% and were ER negative in 62%; findings which are more common in high grade DCIS [4]. In a nested case-control study of 200 patients with DCIS who subsequently developed invasive carcinoma and 474 patients who did not, the statistically significant risk factors associated with the development of invasive carcinoma included HER2 positivity, high expression of cOX2 and the presence of peri-ductal fibrosis [5]. All these studies, and many others, support the conception that DCIS in general and low grade cases in particular do not pose a significant risk to life.

Lobular Carcinoma In Situ (LCIS)

As discussed in Chap. 4 when dealing with in situ lobular neoplasia, it is not clear when to start calling these lesions lobular carcinoma in situ. Perhaps the term can be used in cases which all authors agree that it can be given a score of B5 in a core biopsy, namely pleomorphic cases. In a core biopsy, these casees can look like usual in situ lobular neoplasia at one end (Fig. 5.9) and like high grade DCIS, with comedo necrosis and microcalcification, at the other end (Fig. 5.10). The common feature between them all is the presence of relatively more uniform cells with more uniform nuclei (Figs. 5.9b and 5.10b) but the cells and nuclei are larger than those seen in usual cases of in situ lobular neoplasia, at least 2 times the size of red blood cells, (Fig. 5.9b) and more uniform and dis-cohesive than those seen in high grade DCIS (Fig. 5.10b). Intra cellular mucin may be present (Fig. 5.9b) which is usually absent in high grade DCIS. The presence of these features in cases of high grade in situ lesion should alert the Pathologist to ask for E-cadherin staining which is always negative in these cases (Figs. 5.9c and 5.10c). We usually also ask for ER and HER2 staining which would be useful in confirming the diagnosis if ER is negative and/or HER2 is positive (Fig. 5.9d). In one study, 81% of patients with pleomorphic LCIS presented with fine pleomorphic calcifications on screening mammograms [6].

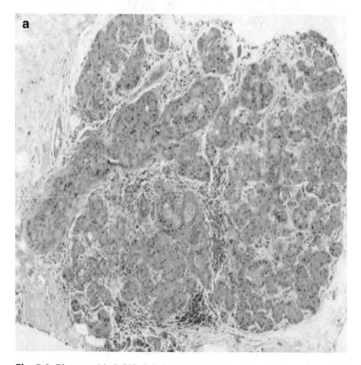

Fig. 5.9 Pleomorphic LCIS (lobular carcinoma in situ): (**a**) Low power; (**b**) High power; (**c**) negative E-Cadherin staining; (**d**) Strongly positive HER2 staining

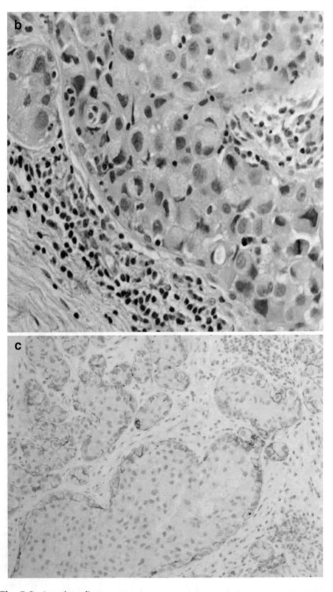

Fig. 5.9 (continued)

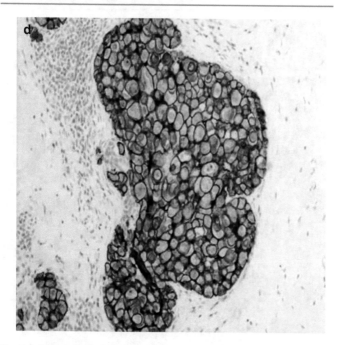

Fig. 5.9 (continued)

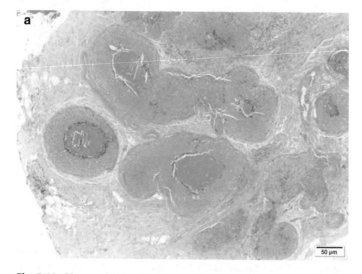

Fig. 5.10 Pleomorphic LCIS with comedo necrosis and microcalcification: (**a**) Low power; (**b**) High power; (**c**) Negative E-Cadherin staining

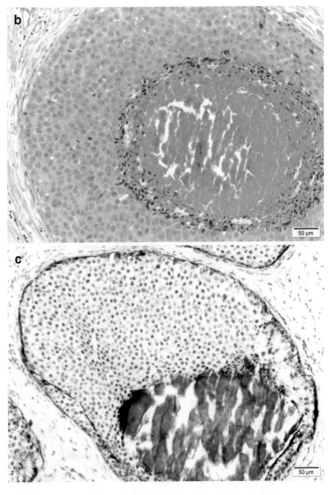

Fig. 5.10 (continued)

As discussed in Chap. 4 another form of in situ lobular neoplasia that an International committee has recommended for category B5a is florid in situ lobular neoplasia, where the whole core biopsy shows closely packed foci of in situ lobular neoplasia of the usual, non-pleomorphic, type; giving an appearance that can simulate low grade DCIS except for the presence of the cellular features of lobular neoplasia [7].

The reason why both theses lobular lesions are given a B5a, instead of B3, is because they are more commonly found, on excision, to be associated with more advanced lesions, commonly an invasive lobular carcinoma, and much less commonly invasive ductal carcinoma or DCIS [8–10]. It is interesting to note that in one of these studies, the invasive tumours that were found with pleomorphic DCIS were all grade 2 or 3, while those associated with florid in situ neoplasia were grade 1 [10].

Paget's Disease of the Nipple

These are usually diagnosed by punch biopsies taken from the nipple because of clinical 'eczematous-like change'. The stratified squamous epithelium covering the nipple contains neoplastic cells, called Paget's cells, quite distinct from the normal squamous cells. Paget cells are larger than the adjacent squamous cell, have a clear cytoplasm and atypical pleomorphic nuclei (Fig. 5.11). The neoplastic cells are usually concentrated at the basal layer of the epidermis but are also seen in other layers. They can be present as single cells or group of cells. There is usually a lymphocytic infiltration, which can be heavy, in the underlying upper dermis. Paget cells stain positively for cytokeratin 7 (Fig. 5.11b) and Cam

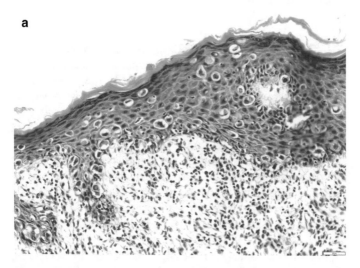

a

Fig. 5.11 Paget's disease o the nipple: (**a**) H&E; (**b**) CK7

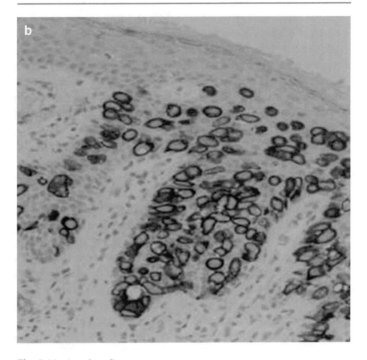

Fig. 5.11 (continued)

5.2. They are positive for HER2 in up to 90% of cases. ER is expressed in around 40% and PR in around 30% of cases [11].

Glandular Paget's disease of the nipple is a rare form of the disease in which the neoplastic cells form glandular structures, usually at the basal part of the epidermis [12] (Fig. 5.12a). Like the usual form of Paget's disease the cells are CK7 and HER2 strongly positive (Fig. 5.12b).

Pigmented Paget's disease of the nipple is another rare variant of the disease that can mimic malignant melanoma both clinically and microscopically [13]. In this condition, the clear cytoplasm of Paget cells contain phagocytosed brown melanin pigments, but the cells stain positive for CK7 and negative for melanoma markers like S100 and HMB-45.

Even in the absence of melanin granules in the cytoplasm, Paget's disease of the nipple has to be differentiated from malig-

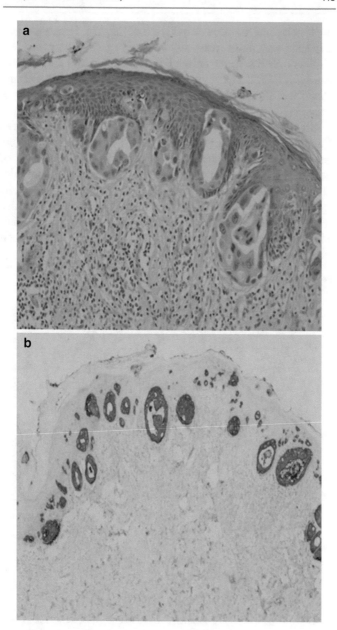

Fig. 5.12 Glandular Paget's disease o the nipple: (**a**) H&E; (**b**) HER2

nant melanoma and Bowen's disease of the skin. Hence, we usually stain sections of cases suspected of Paget's disease for CK7, S100 and HER2. Paget's disease is positive for CK7 and, in most cases, for HER2. Melanomas would be positive for S100 and negative for CK7 and HER2. Bowen's disease of the skin would be negative for all three markers.

Staining for HER2 is also useful in differentiating Paget cells from Toker cells [14]. These are clear cells present within the stratified squamous epithelium of the nipple of around 11% of women [15]. Toker cells, like Paget's cells, have a cytoplasm paler than the surrounding keratinocytes, but differ from Paget's cells by being smaller and having bland nuclei. They are CK7 positive (Fig. 5.13), but HER2 negative. It has been suggested that Toker cells are derived from sebaceous glands rather than from ductal epithelium as is the case with Paget cells [15].

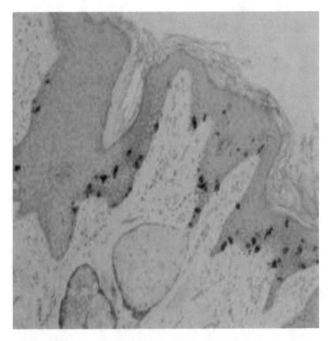

Fig. 5.13 Toker cells staining positive with CK7

Paget's disease of the nipple is essentially an in situ carcinoma where the malignant cells are confined to the basement membrane of the epidermis. Rare cases of invasive Paget's disease have been described where the neoplastic cells have penetrated the basement membrane and invaded the underlying dermis usually to a very limited extent [16]. In the latter study there was a direct relationship between the horizontal extent of Paget's disease and the presence of invasion [16]. Invasive Paget's disease has to be differentiated from invasion of the nipple epidermis by an underlying invasive cancer which can be of any histological type.

Paget's disease of the nipple is associated with an underlying carcinoma, in more than 90% of patients. The underlying lesion is usually a high grade HER2 positive DCIS which is sometimes seen in continuity with the malignant cells within the epidermis. Some cases may be associated with an invasive ductal carcinoma which can be present deep in the breast. I have never seen Paget's disease in association with invasive lobular carcinoma, but I have seen a case where there were two underlying invasive carcinoma, one ductal and the other mucinous. All lesions wee HER2 positive.

Intracystic and Solid Papillary Carcinomas

There is a great deal of confusion about the nomenclature, criteria for diagnosis and behaviour of these lesions and whether they are in situ or invasive tumours. The current consensus, which is in itself confusing, is that they are 'indolent invasive tumours' but should be managed as in situ carcinomas unless they are associated with clear evidence of invasion [17]. Hence, if they are not associated with clear invasive elements the are given a score of ab5a when seen in a core biopsy.

All lesions are relatively large rounded well defined and show extensive 'papillary' proliferation of uniform CK5 negative ER strongly positive neoplastic epithelial cells. Most lesions are surrounded by condensed layers of fibrous tissue 'capsule'. The papillary architecture can be obvious in the form of arborizing fronds within a dilated cyst (Fig. 5.14, intracystic papillary carcinoma), but in many cases the papillary architecture is subtle and can only be realised because of the presence of small islands of vascular

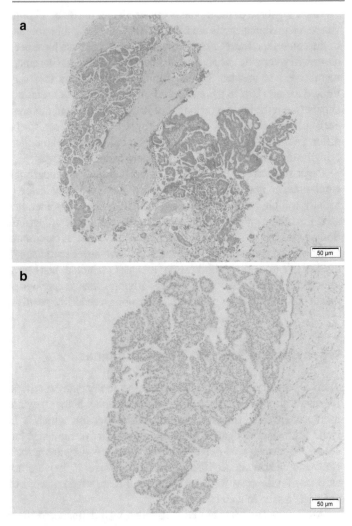

Fig. 5.14 Intracystic papillary carcinoma in a core biopsy: (**a**) H&E; (**b**) negative staining with CK5

fibrous tissue between the proliferating cells which are presumed to represent 'fused' papillae. The lesion will thus appear solid (Fig. 5.15) or sometimes show a cribriform pattern. The neoplastic cells in some solid lesions may show features of neuroendocrine differentiation, in the form of spindle shaped cells and positive staining for neuroendocrine granules like chromogranin, synaptophysin (Fig. 5.15d) or CD56, or show mucin production. Lesions with these latter features can form multiple closely packed structures that fit with each other like a jigsaw, and it has been suggested that such cases should be considered invasive [18].

Different names have been given to these lesions that do not help to differentiate them from each other. The terms encysted and encapsulated can be applied to all as all are supposed to be arising within cysts and most have a surrounding fibrous tissue capsule. The term solid papillary carcinoma is currently restricted to lesions that show neuroendocrine differentiation or mucin production, but there are solid cases with no such differentiation. It may be easier to classify the cases into two main categories:

- intracystic papillary carcinoma where the papillary fronds are still obvious, and
- solid where such fronds are not obvious. Then subdivide the latter cases into two
  - solid papillary
  - and solid papillary with neuroendocrine differentiation or mucus production, with the understanding that the latter type can be multiple and sometimes is seen in the form of closely packed foci.

Although the great majority of intracystic and solid papillary carcinomas have low grade nuclei and are ER positive, rare ER negative cases with high grade nuclei and increased mitotic activity have been reported. These are thought to be more aggressive and frequently show evidence of stromal invasion [19].

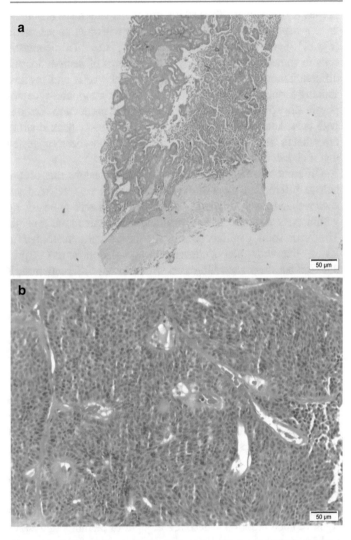

Fig. 5.15 Solid papillary carcinoma in a core biopsy: (**a**) H&E; (**b**) High power showing islands of vascular fibrous tissue between the solid proliferation of the neoplastic cells; (**c**) negative CK5 staining; (**d**) the neuroendocrine variant of solid papillary carcinoma showing positive staining with synaptophysin

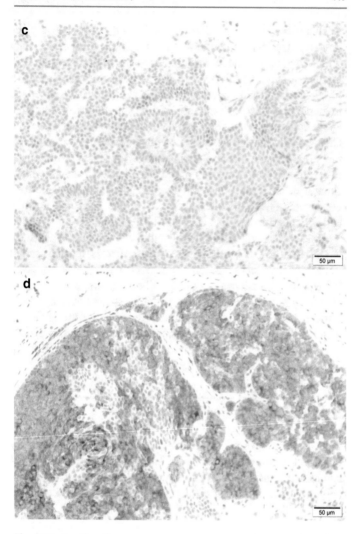

Fig. 5.15 (continued)

In practice, once a papillary lesion is seen in a core biopsy, the first step would be to decide whether the lesion is benign, benign with atypia or malignant. Benign lesions are more common than malignant and as described in Chap. 4 consist of thin fronds of fibrous tissue usually covered by two layers of cells, luminal and myoepithelial. Hyperplasia, in the form of more than two luminal epithelial layers, may be present. When hyperplasia is present, a CK5 staining may be needed to confirm the presence of myoepithelial cells in the lesion. In benign papillary lesions with atypia, in addition to the presence of atypical nuclei, CK5 staining might show wide areas of CK5 negativity. In contrast, malignant lesions are devoid of CK5 positive cells except for the occasional positive cell at the periphery (Figs. 5.14b and 5.15c).

Once the lesion is identified as malignant, the next step is to try to classify it. If there are obvious papillary fronds, it can be called intracystic papillary carcinoma (Fig. 5.14a). If the lesion appears to be solid with islands of vascular fibrous tissue, immunohistochemistry for an endocrine marker, like synaptophysin, would separate the solid lesions with no neuroendocrine differentiation, which are more common, from the lesions with such differentiation. Staining for ER is also advisable to detect the rare ER negative cases that are thought to be more aggressive.

Invasive Lesions (B5b)

Most invasive lesions seen in breast core biopsies are primary invasive breast carcinomas. Much less common are primary sarcomas and lymphomas and rarely metastatic lesions from extramammary sites including metastatic carcinomas and sarcomas.

Primary Invasive Breast Carcinoma

A diagnosis of invasive breast carcinoma in a core biopsy should provide information about the morphological type, the grade of the tumour, the presence or absence of associated DCIS and microcalcification, as well as the oestrogen and progesterone receptor and HER2 status. Additional information that can be useful, particularly in ER negative tumours, are the presence or absence of necrosis and the degree of stromal lymphocytic infiltration. Retraction artefacts in a core biopsy can be easily confused with lymphatic invasion, hence, the presence of lympho-vascular invasion in a core biopsy should not be mentioned in the report unless there is strong evidence of its presence in the form of definite tumour cells present in a well-defined vascular structures, preferably in association with an adjacent vein, nerve or a small capillary.

Morphological Types

For invasive tumours, most of the special histological types, e.g. tubular, invasive cribriform and mucinous carry a better prognosis than the usual invasive ductal and lobular types. For this reason the strict criteria for the diagnosis of these special types should be followed. For example, for the diagnosis of pure tubular or cribriform carcinoma more than 90% of the tumour should be composed of well-formed tubules or cribriform structures, respectively. Similarly, for the diagnosis of pure mucinous carcinoma, 90% of the tumour must exhibit the typical mucinous appearance. However, if the tumour is composed of a mixture of tubules and cribriform structures, it has to be called tubular if tubules compose more than 50% of the lesion, and cribriform otherwise.

Mixed types do occur, but there are also strict rules for diagnosing mixed tumours. For example, for mixed tubular/ductal or tubular/lobular, the tubular elements should comprise between 75 and 90% of the surface area of the tumour sections examined. In mixed mucinous/ductal tumours, the mucinous areas should comprise 10–90% of the tumour. Similarly, in mixed ductal/lobular, the ductal elements should form between 10 and 90% of the tumour. The Pathologist should also be alert to spot the uncommon non-epithelial malignant tumours, e.g. lymphomas, angiosarcomas and other soft tissue sarcomas and to be able to differentiate the latter from metaplastic carcinomas using keratin immunostains. Following is a brief description of some of the special types of invasive breast carcinoma.

Invasive Ductal Carcinoma

Most primary invasive breast carcinomas are the lesions most widely known as invasive ductal carcinoma. These are sometimes called invasive ductal carcinoma, not otherwise specified (NOS), or simply Not otherwise specified carcinoma. This is to distinguish them from other, less common, types of primary breast cancers that have specific feature like mucin production for mucinous carcinoma or well-formed tubular structures for tubular carcinoma. However, for practical purposes the term invasive ductal carcinoma, or its abbreviation as IDC, is the one used by most Pathologists as well as Breast Surgeons and Oncologists and in most scientific publications.

The tumour cells in invasive ductal carcinoma can be arranged in tubular structures or in solid groups or sheets of variable sizes or in a combination of all these forms (Fig. 5.16). Small areas where the tumour cells are arranged in single files may be occasionally seen. Like all other types of invasive breast carcinoma, the tumours are graded according to the percentage of tubule formation, the degree of nuclear pleomorphism and mitotic activity (see below). The stroma can be scanty or abundant or described as desmoplastic

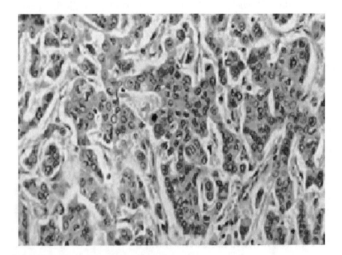

Fig. 5.16 Invasive ductal carcinoma

where abundant proliferating fibroblasts intervene between tumour cells. This might give rise to a characteristic stellate radiological appearance. Most cases however present clinically or radiologically as solid masses. The tumours can be grade 1, 2 or 3. Stromal elastosis and microcalcifications are more common in low grade tumours which are usually ER and PR positive, HER2 negative, while necrosis and stromal lymphocytic infiltration are more common in high grade lesions, particularly ER negative ones.

Pleomorphic Invasive Ductal Carcinoma

These are rare tumours characterised by the presence of marked nuclear pleomorphism (>6 fold variation of nuclear size), in more than 50% of tumour cells, as well as numerous multinucleated tumour giant cells [1, 2] (Fig. 5.17). In a series of 37 cases the age incidence was 23–78 years. The tumours were mostly well-defined and varied in size between 1.2 and 11.6 cm. Necrosis was present in 76% of cases and positive axillary nodes were present in 52% [20, 21]. Around a third of the tumours had a spindle cell component and a third had associated DCIS [20, 21]. ER and PR

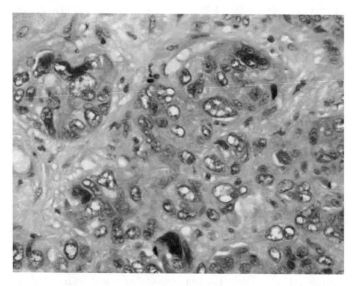

Fig. 5.17 Pleomorphic invasive ductal carcinoma

were negative in 94–100% and HER2 was negative in 40–84% [20–22]. Five-year survival was 38% if there are spindle cell element and 89% in the absence of spindle cell elements [21]. The case illustrated here (Fig. 5.17) was seen in a patient with Huntington's disease who died 14 months after presentation [23].

Invasive Lobular Carcinoma

This is the second most common histological type of breast carcinoma with an estimated incidence of around 7% of all histological types [24, 25]. Radiologically, the lesions commonly present as spiculated masses or architectural distortions [26]. This is reflected in the ill-defined margins of these lesions as seen grossly and microscopically, which lead to higher rates of margin involvement in cases treated by conservative surgery [24, 25]. Multi-centricity is also thought to be a feature of these lesions, although its incidence in large series is only marginally higher than that noted in invasive ductal carcinoma.

The tumour is characterised microscopically by the presence of distinctive monomorphic tumour cells with pale-stained cytoplasm and rounded dark-stained nuclei. Classically the cells are arranged in single files (Fig. 5.18) and targetoid patterns around normal ducts, separated by abundant fibrous tissue. Less commonly the cells may be arranged in alveolar patterns of 20 cells or more (Fig. 5.19), in trabeculae (Fig. 5.20) or in larger solid sheets, giving rise, respectively, to the alveolar, trabecular and solid variant of invasive lobular carcinoma. Other subtypes include those with abundant intracellular mucin giving rise to the signet ring variant and those with individual cells having abundant cytoplasm with relatively small nuclei, similar to histiocytes, giving rise to the rare 'histiocytoid' variant (Fig. 5.21). Lastly, the pleomorphic variant is characterised by the presence of high grade nuclei, at least 2 times the size of a red blood cell (Fig. 5.22). Foci of in situ lobular carcinoma may or may not be present in association with the invasive tumour.

All variants have two features in common, the characteristic morphology of the neoplastic cells and the absence of E-Cadherin membrane staining. As described above, the tumour cells are monomorphic with pale-stained cytoplasm and rounded dark-

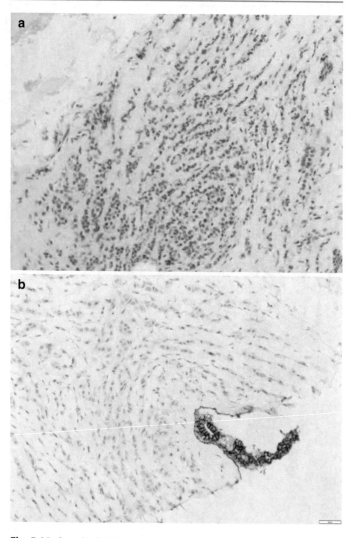

Fig. 5.18 Invasive lobular carcinoma, classical variant: (**a**) H&E; (**b**) negative E-Cadherin staining

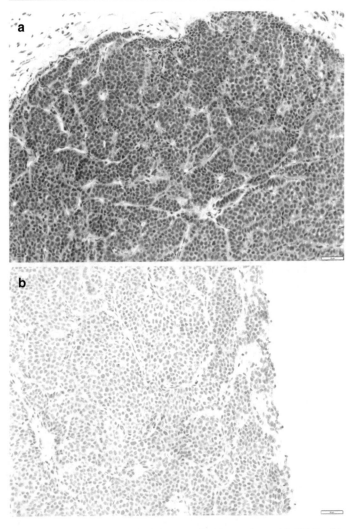

Fig. 5.19 Invasive lobular carcinoma, alveolar variant: (**a**) H&E; (**b**) E-Cadherin; (**c**) ER (**d**) Synaptophysin negative

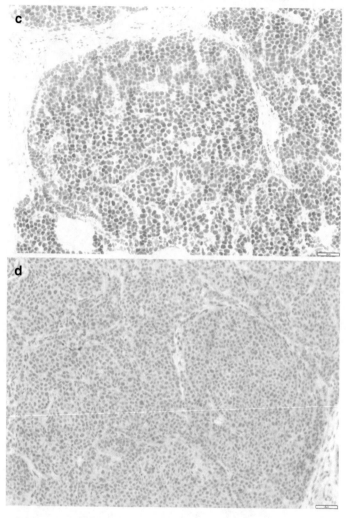

Fig. 5.19 (continued)

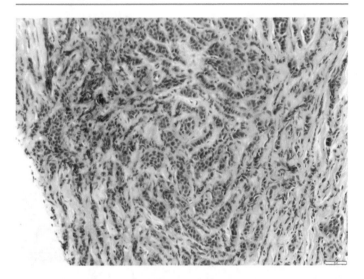

Fig. 5.20 Invasive lobular carcinoma, trabecular variant

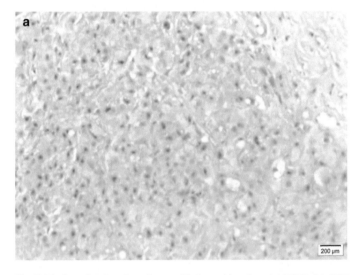

Fig. 5.21 Invasive ductal carcinoma, histiocytoid variant: (**a**) H&E; (**b**) CK7

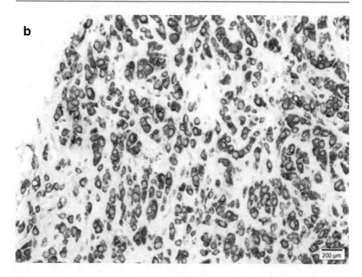

Fig. 5.21 (continued)

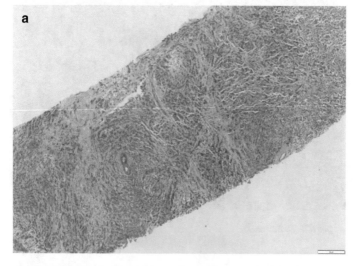

Fig. 5.22 Pleomorphic invasive lobular carcinoma: (**a**) low power view of a core biopsy, (**b**) high power; (**c**) E-Cadherin negative, the tumour cells are arranged in a targetoid pattern around an E-cadherin positively stained normal duct

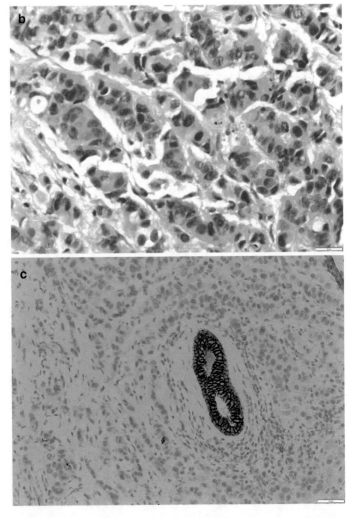

Fig. 5.22 (continued)

stained nuclei. Intracellular mucin may be evident. However, around 5% the classical, single file, variant are E-cadherin positive in spite of the presence of all the other morphological and molecular features characteristic of lobular carcinoma. Most invasive lobular carcinomas are ER and PR positive (Fig. 5.23) and HER2 negative. They are also GATA3 positive (Fig. 5.24). Rare ER negative HER2 positive cases do occur (Fig. 5.25) and most of these are of the pleomorphic variant. The tumours are usually grade 2, but the pleomorphic variant can be grade 2 or 3.

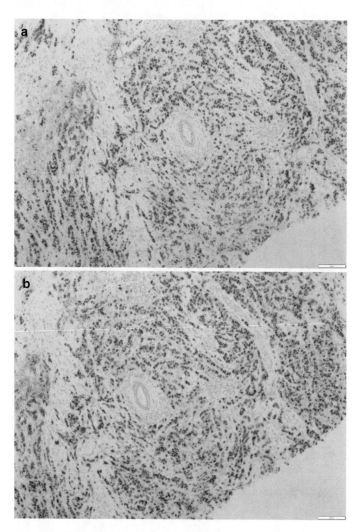

Fig. 5.23 Invasive lobular carcinoma: (**a**) ER positive; (**b**) PR positive

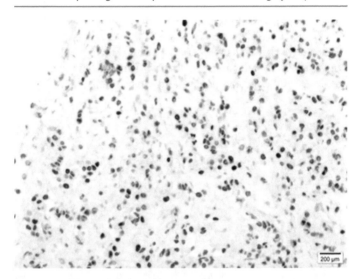

Fig. 5.24 Invasive lobular carcinoma, positive GATA3 staining

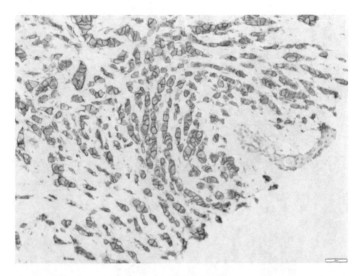

Fig. 5.25 Invasive lobular carcinoma, HER2 positive

In core biopsies, the lobular nature of the classical variant with single file pattern is usually quiet obvious and might not need confirmation by staining for E-cadherin. In fact some authors advise not to do E-cadherin for such cases to avoid confusion if they prove to be positive as is the case in around 5% of cases. However, in our institution we usually stain such cases for E-Cadherin to confirm the diagnosis as some cases of invasive ductal carcinoma may show areas of single filing and these together with the rest of the tumour will be E-Cadherin positive. In the rare case of classical invasive lobular carcinoma that proves to be E-cadherin positive we usually qualify the diagnosis by calling the tumour E-Cadherin positive invasive carcinoma with classical lobular pattern. The case will be managed as invasive lobular carcinoma which usually necessitates bilateral investigation of the breasts by MRI to exclude, or prove, the presence of other foci of the tumour.

In the non-classical variants of invasive lobular carcinoma, the suspicion that the lesion could be of lobular phenotype is usually aroused by the presence of the typical lobular cellular morphology described above, and it is essential in these cases to confirm the diagnosis by demonstrating the absence of E-Cadherin membrane staining. In this respect, it must be added here that other morphological types of poorly differentiated breast carcinomas, particularly high grade ductal and metaplastic carcinomas, may show diminished or absence of E-Cadherin membrane staining, but the morphology of such lesions is quite different and in practice does not call for E-Cadherin staining.

The classical type of invasive lobular carcinoma, where the tumour cells are arranged in single files and small groups widely separated by fibrous tissue, can sometimes give a deceptively benign appearance particularly when the neoplastic cells are relatively few. The presence of cells arranged in rows with enlarged hyperchromatic nuclei should raise suspicion, and immunohistochemistry, using a wide spectrum cytokeratin stain, carried out for confirmation. Lymphoid aggregates and follicles are commonly seen in association with invasive lobular carcinoma.

On the other hand, lymphocytes may be sometimes seen arranged in rows thus mimicking lobular carcinoma, but lymphocytes will be negative with the cytokeratin stain. Also, some areas in sclerosing adenosis may appear as a single row of epithelial cells, but their presence in an otherwise typical focus of sclerosing adenosis, should prevent a misdiagnosis of invasive carcinoma.

Invasive Tubular Carcinoma

In tubular carcinoma, the glands may be angulated with tapering ends, and they are irregularly scattered within a fibrous stroma, which may be desmoplastic (Fig. 5.26). The glands have wide lumina, which are sometimes multiple. The cells are usually slightly larger than normal ductal cells, have vesicular nuclei and small cytoplasmic protrusions into the lumen (snouts). The neoplastic glands are relatively abundant, compared with those seen in the centre of a radial scar, which is one of the main differential diagnosis particularly in small lesions. Commonly, there are associated foci of low grade, cribriform, DCIS, from which neoplastic glands may appear to be budding out. Columnar change may be also present. Myoepithelial cells are absent as seen in H&E stained sections, as well as in sections stained immunohistochemically for myoepithelial markers like smooth muscle actin, p63 (Fig. 5.26b) or CD10. In actin-stained sections, caution must

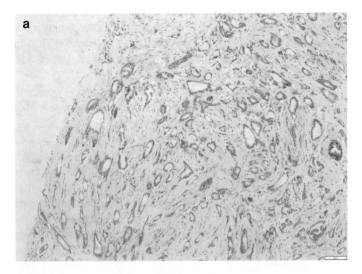

Fig. 5.26 Invasive tubular carcinoma: (**a**) H&E; (**b**) p63; (**c**) ER

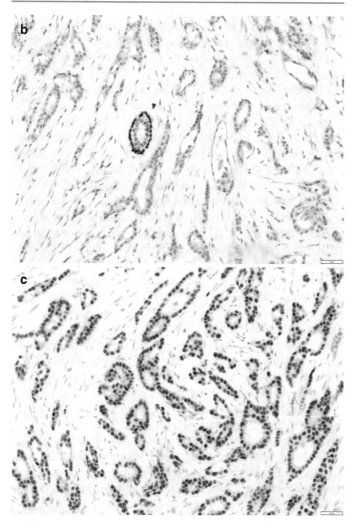

Fig. 5.26 (continued)

be taken not to interpret compressed myofibroblasts around ducts as myoepithelial cells.

Tubular carcinoma can be seen mixed with other morphological types of breast carcinoma, particularly with invasive ductal carcinoma. The diagnosis of pure tubular carcinoma is usually made when at least 90% of the tumour cells are arranged in the characteristic tubular pattern. The tumour is considered of mixed type when the tubular elements are present in 50–90% of the tumour surface area.

The incidence of tubular carcinoma has increased since the introduction of mammographic screening, and most lesions detected by this method are usually of small size, being mostly less than 10 mm in maximum dimension [27, 28]. The tumours are usually grade 1 and almost always ER and PR positive (Fig. 5.26c) and HER2 negative. The intensity of ER and PR staining can be sometimes less than that noted in well differentiated ER positive invasive ductal carcinoma [29]. Involvement of axillary nodes is rare and is only seen occasionally in tumours larger than 10 mm [27]. Prognosis of pure tubular carcinomas after excision is excellent with reported 5 and 10 year disease free survival of 96 and 89% respectively, and 5 and 10 year overall survival 98 and 92% respectively [30]. The prognosis of mixed types is less favourable.

Invasive Cribriform Carcinoma

These are rarely seen on their own, but occur more commonly mixed with tubular carcinomas [31–33]. Unlike cribriform DCIS, the outlines of the lesions' components are irregular (Fig. 5.27) and there are no surrounding myoepithelial cells (Fig. 5.27b, c). Like tubular carcinomas, they are usually grade 1, ER and PR positive (Fig. 5.27d) and HER2 negative. In its pure form, the cribriform pattern is present in at least 90% of the lesion. The lesion is also considered pure cribriform if up to 50% of the lesion consists of tubular elements. Pure invasive cribriform carcinoma has good prognosis with rare axillary lymph node or distal metastasis [34].

Invasive Mucinous Carcinoma

These are tumours characterised by the presence of abundant extra-cellular mucin (Fig. 5.28a–c). The tumours are usually grade 1 or 2 and mostly ER and PR positive (Fig. 5.28d), HER2 negative. Rare HER2 positive cases do occur (Fig. 5.28e). Sixty per cent of invasive mucinous carcinomas are WT1 positive ([35]; Fig. 5.28f).

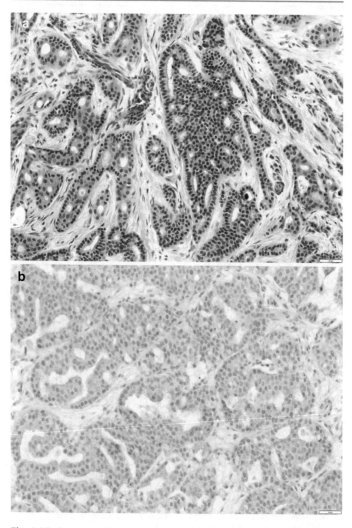

Fig. 5.27 Invasive cribriform carcinoma: (**a**) H&E; (**b**) p63; (**c**) CK5; (**d**) ER

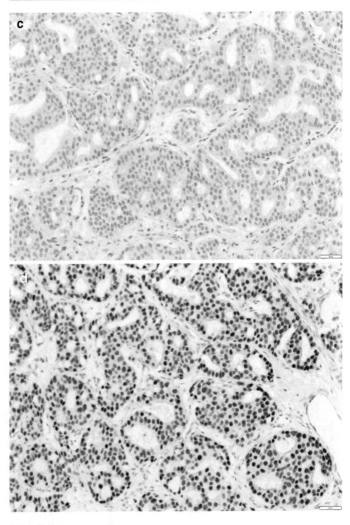

Fig. 5.27 (continued)

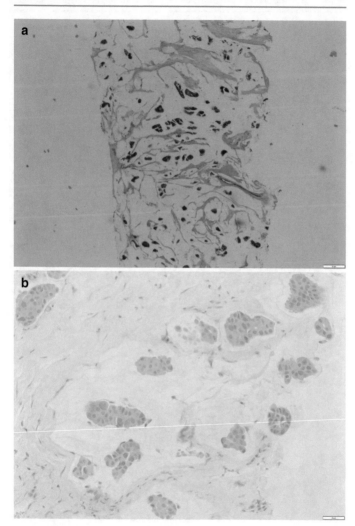

Fig. 5.28 Invasive mucinous carcinoma… (**a**) low power of a core biopsy; (**b**) high power; (**c**) Alcian blue/PAS mucin stain; (**d**) ER; (**e**) HER2 positive; (**f**) WT1 positive

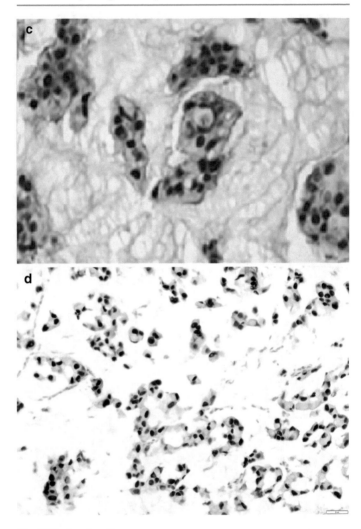

Fig. 5.28 (continued)

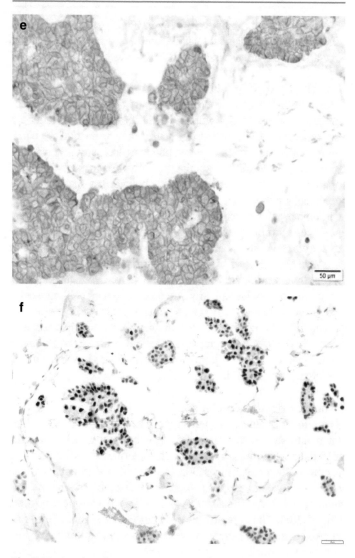

Fig. 5.28 (continued)

They are indolent tumours with low incidence of axillary node or distal metastasis. The estimated 5 and 10 year disease free and overall survival are around 92 and 75% respectively [30].

Lympho-Epithelioma-Like Carcinoma

This is a histological type of breast carcinoma characterised by the presence of a heavy lymphocytic infiltrate [36]. The latter can be sometimes so heavy that it obscures the presence of the carcinoma cells (Fig. 5.29). The lymphocytes lack any atypical features and on careful examination small islands of atypical epithelial cells can be identified and confirmed as such by immunohistochemistry staining for cytokeratns markers. Medullary carcinomas of the breast can be also heavily infiltrated with lymphocytes but not to that extent. Also, unlike medullary carcinomas, lympho-epithelioma like carcinoma can be ER positive or negative (Fig. 5.29d). A core biopsy with a heavy lymphocytic infiltrate and no obvious epithelial elements, necessitates a stain for cytokeratin to identify any obscured malignant epithelial cells, and if these are absent, lymphoma markers have to be carried out to help differentiating reactive from neoplastic lymphocytic infiltrates. In contrast with lympho-epithelioma of the head and neck, there is no evidence to implicate Epstein-Barr virus infection in the breast version [36].

Invasive Apocrine Carcinoma

The tumour architecture in this type of carcinoma is usually similar to invasive ductal carcinoma, but the tumour cells have the abundant eosinophilc cytoplasm characteristic of other apocrine lesions of the breast (Fig. 5.30a, b). Immunohistochemically, like other benign and atypical apocrine lesions of the breast, the tumour is ER and PR negative and GCDFP-15 strongly positive (Fig. 5.30c). They are also positive for GATA3 (Fig. 5.30d) and androgen receptors, and we have found out that they are also positive for Claudin 1 and 3 (Fig. 5.30e, f) and negative for claudin 4 [37]. The tumours can be HER2 positive or negative. In a study of 38 cases of pure invasive apocrine carcinomas, where at least 90% of the tumour shows apocrine differentiation, HER2 was amplified

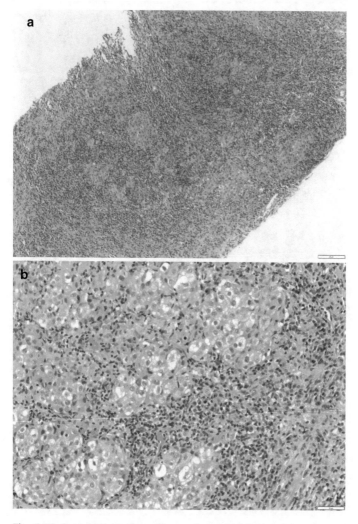

Fig. 5.29 Lympho-epithelioma-like carcinoma: (**a**) Low power of a core biopsy; (**b**) high power; (**c**) Cam 5.2 showing positive staining of the malignant cells; (**d**) ER positive

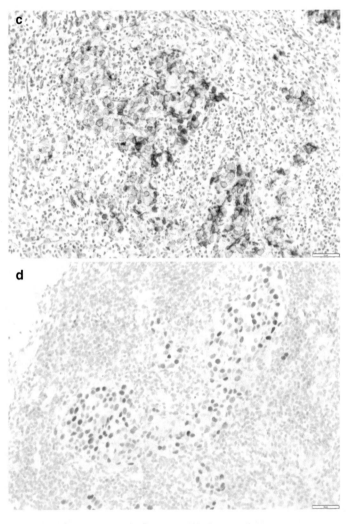

Fig. 5.29 (continued)

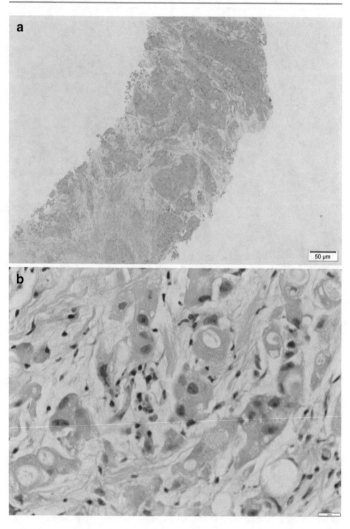

Fig. 5.30 Invasive apocrine carcinoma: (**a**) Low power view of a core biopsy; (**b**) high power; (**c**) Strong GCDFP-15 positive staining; (**d**) positive GATA3 staining; (**e**) positive Claudin 1 staining; (**f**) positive Claudin 3

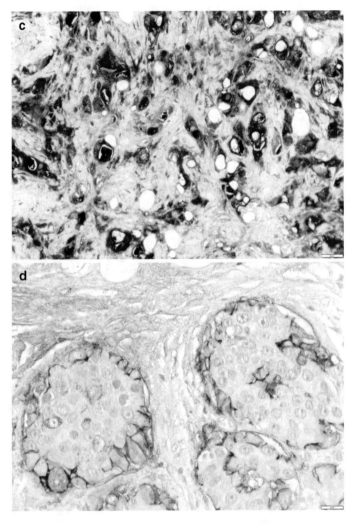

Fig. 5.30 (continued)

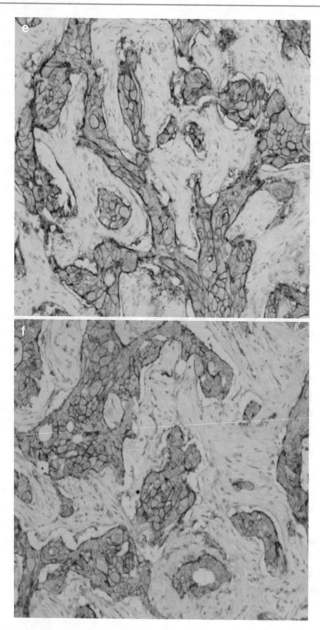

Fig. 5.30 (continued)

in 54% of cases [38], which means that around half apocrine carcinomas are triple negative. Patients with pure apocrine carcinoma seem to have worse prognosis than patients with invasive ductal carcinoma as regards disease free survival, but not overall survival [39]. They also seem to have an increased risk of developing contra lateral carcinoma [39].

Invasive Papillary Carcinoma

This is an extremely rare breast tumour [40]. It can occur on its own or in association with intracystic or solid papillary carcinoma. The tumour cells are arranged in interconnected glandular structures with short papillary projections with no significant intervening stroma (Fig. 5.31). Nuclear pleomorphism is usually moderate or high and the few tumours I have seen, including the one seen in Fig. 5.31, were all triple negative. There are no available data about the prognosis of the disease.

Invasive Micropapillary Carcinoma

These are relatively more common than the above type and can occur in a pure form or mixed with invasive ductal elements. In a study of 1056 cases of breast carcinomas, the micropapillary pattern was noted in 51 tumours (around 5%). This was less than 25% in 9 cases (18%), between 25 and 49% in 11 cases (22%), between 50 and 75% in 12 cases (24%) and more than 75% in 19 cases (37%) [41]. A case is considered a pure invasive micropapillary carcinoma if the micropapillary component is more than 75% of the lesion [42].

The tumour cells are arranged in clusters devoid of fibrovascular cores and situated within empty stromal spaces ([42]; Fig. 5.32). The cells are arranged with their luminal surfaces projecting outwards rather than inwards, giving rise to an 'inside-out' pattern that can be better visualised by epithelial markers like CAM 5.2 and EMA (Fig. 5.32c, d). E-Cadherin is absent at the new outer surface of the neoplastic cells (Fig. 5.32e), possibly indicating a disturbance in the cell adhesion molecules [43].

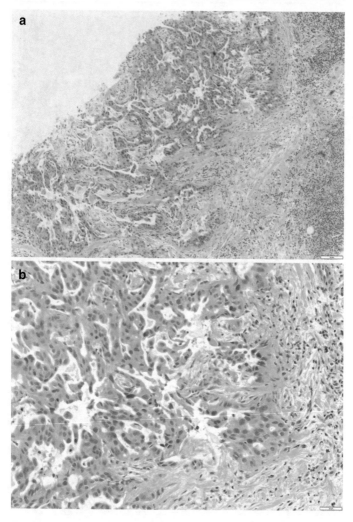

Fig. 5.31 Invasive papillary carcinoma: (**a**) low power; (**b**) high power view

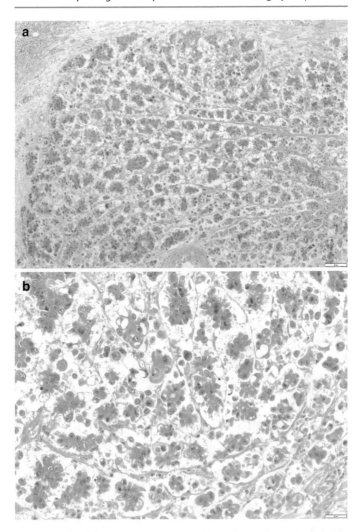

Fig. 5.32 Invasive micropapillary carcinoma: (**a**) low power; (**b**) high power view showing the tumour clusters surrounded by empty spaces; (**c**) Cam 5.2 staining of a normal duct showing positively stained luminal surface; (**d**) Cam 5.2 staining of micropapillary carcinoma showing reversal of the staining to the outer surface of the tumour clusters; (**e**) E-Cadherin staining

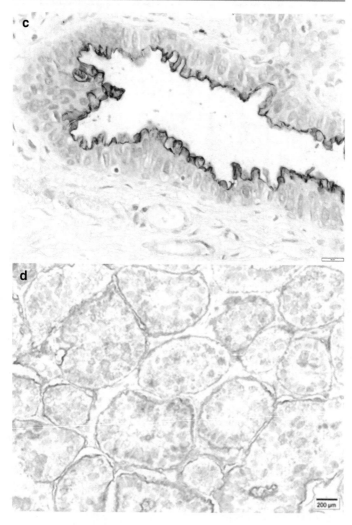

Fig. 5.32 (continued)

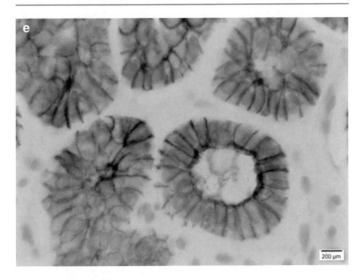

Fig. 5.32 (continued)

Invasive micropapillary carcinoma is considered an aggressive tumour. In a study of 62 cases, 34 (87%) were grade 3, focal or massive lymphatic permeation was present in 39 (63%) and axillary lymph node metastases in 56 (90%) [43]. In that study 32% were ER positive, 20% PR positive and 95% HER2 positive. Of 29 patients with follow up information, 71% had local recurrence and 49% died of the disease. The percentage of the micropapillary pattern in the tumour does not seem to be related to the presence of lymph node metastasis [41, 42].

In invasive micropapillary mucinous carcinoma, the spaces around the cell tufts are occupied by mucin, but it is not clear whether this type of tumour is a variant of micropapillary or of mucinous carcinoma [42].

Neuroendocrine Tumours of the Breast

Neuroendocrine granules as demonstrated by immunohistochemistry, e.g. chromogranin, synaptophysin or CD56, are seen in up to 30% of invasive breast carcinomas [44]. Their presence is not considered enough to call the case a neuroendocrine tumour, the tumour should also have a 'neuroendocrine morphology' similar to that seen in neuroendocrine tumours of the gastrointestinal tract and lung [44]. There is no specific threshold for neuroendocrine marker positivity. Three histological subtypes are described [44]:

1. **Neuroendocrine tumours, well differentiated (carcinoid-like)**

   The cells may be polyhedral or spindle shaped and are arranged in well-defined clusters. The nuclei are of low or intermediate grade and are ER strongly positive. This helps differentiating them from metastatic carcinoid tumours arising in the gastro-intestinal tract or lung.

2. **Neuroendocrine carcinoma, poorly differentiated/Small cell carcinoma**

   These are similar to small cell carcinoma of the lung and can be TTF1 positive (Fig. 5.33), hence thorough investigation of the lung, thyroid, liver and G.I and biliary tracts have to be carried out before confirming a primary breast origin. The few cases we saw were triple negative and showed weak GATA3 expression (Fig. 5.33d).

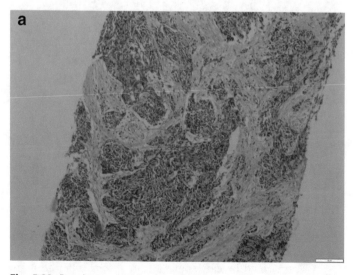

Fig. 5.33 Invasive neuroendocrine carcinoma, poorly differentiated: (**a**) Low power view of a core biopsy; (**b**) high power; (**c**) TTF1 positive

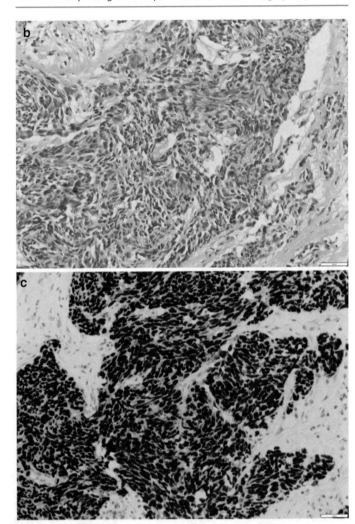

Fig. 5.33 (continued)

3. **Invasive breast carcinoma with neuroendocrine differenti-ation, where focal 'carcinoid-like areas' are present**

 These could be carcinomas of no special type that show focal 'carcinoid like areas' as well as positive staining with neuroendocrine markers (Fig. 5.34). The case illustrated here

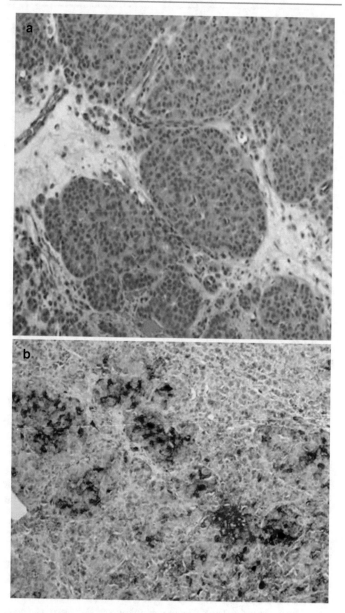

Fig. 5.34 Invasive breast carcinoma with neuroendocrine differentiation; (**a**) H&E; (**b**) Chromogranin positivity; (**c**) ER positive

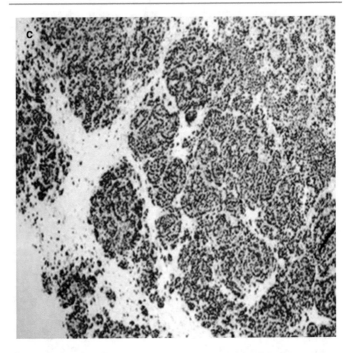

Fig. 5.34 (continued)

was ER strongly positive (Fig. 5.34c). Also included in this group are the hypercellular variant of invasive mucinous carcinoma and the invasive form of solid papillary carcinoma [44].

There are conflicting reports in the literature as regards the prognosis of these lesions, possibly because of the small numbers studied and variation in definition; but it seems that the poorly differentiated variant has a worse prognosis than the other two variants [45].

Glycogen-Rich Clear Cell Carcinoma

This is defined as a carcinoma in which more than 90% of the tumour cells have abundant clear cytoplasm containing glycogen as can be demonstrated by PAS stain (Fig. 5.35). The tumour can be in situ or invasive [46]. The invasive tumour cells grow in solid nests, cords or sheets. The presence of tubular structures seems to be exceptionally uncommon [46]. A recent analysis of 155 invasive cases from the US Surveillance, Epidemiology and End Results (SEER) programme database, suggested that this rare type of breast carcinoma is more likely to be high grade, triple

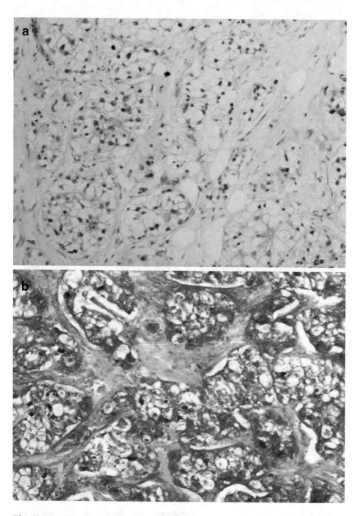

Fig. 5.35 Glycogen-rich clear cell carcinoma: (**a**) H&E; (**b**) PAS stain; (**c**) Diastase-PAS stain

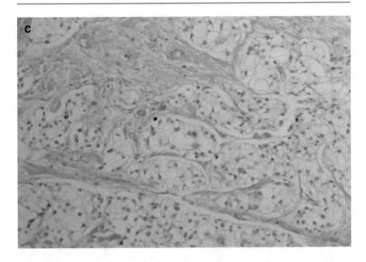

Fig. 5.35 (continued)

negative and more aggressive than other types of breast carcinoma irrespective of age, stage, grade and treatment [47].

Lipid-Rich Carcinoma

A few cases of invasive breast carcinomas with lipid-rich neoplastic cells have been described in the literature [48]. The cells have clear cytoplasm which does not stain with PAS, but are positively stained with Sudan III in frozen sections. The tumour cells are arranged in solid sheets of variable sizes. In a study of 17 cases the cells were negative for ER, CK 5/6, CK14, S100 and p63 but positive for HER2 and one was positive for PR [48].

Triple Negative Invasive Breast Carcinoma

This is a group of invasive breast carcinomas characterised by the absence of ER and PR expression and HER2 gene amplification. Most of the tumours in this group have a more aggressive behaviour than the more common types of breast carcinomas discussed above, but there are some types including the salivary gland-like tumours and low grade adenosquamous carcinoma, which are indolent and have a good prognosis. As the whole group lack ER expression and HER2 amplification, they are not suitable for adjuvant treatment with anti-oestrogen or anti-HER2 medications respectively, and therefor chemotherapy or other newly developed targeted medications are used. The group can be divided into the following subgroups:

1. **Triple negative invasive ductal carcinoma**

    Most of these tumours have a morphology that cannot be distinguished from ER positive or HER2 positive invasive ductal carcinomas. However, two variants of these tumours have peculiar microscopic appearances that would suggest their triple negativity once they have been examined microscopically:

    (a) <u>**Ring-like carcinoma**</u>, where the tumour cells are arranged in a ring manner around a large central area of necrosis and fibrosis (Fig. 5.36).

    (b) <u>**Invasive carcinomas with comedo-like necrosis**</u>, where the tumour cells are arranged in solid groups or trabeculae separated by wide areas of structureless, comedo-like necrosis (Fig. 5.37)

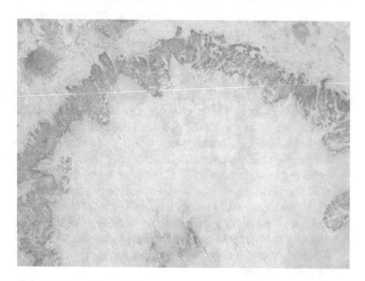

Fig. 5.36 Ring-like carcinoma

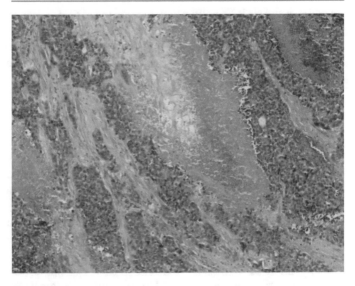

Fig. 5.37 Invasive carcinoma with comedo-like necrosis

2. **Medullary and Medullary-like carcinoma**

For diagnosing medullary carcinoma, the tumour should consist of markedly pleomorphic cells arranged in solid, syncytial, interconnected sheets with well-defined, pushing margins, minimal intratumoural stroma and heavy infiltration with lymphocytes (Fig. 5.38). DCIS elements are usually absent, and the tumour is ER, PR and HER2 negative. If any of these criteria is not met, the tumour can be called invasive ductal carcinoma with medullary features, atypical medullary or medullary-like carcinoma. These lesions are more common in pre-menopausal patients with BRCA1 gene mutation and it is estimated that around 25% of patients with medullary or medullary-like carcinomas have this particular gene mutation. As a core biopsy will only show a small part of the lesion, the full criteria for making a diagnosis of medullary carcinoma are almost always impossible to establish and a more reasonable diagnosis would be a grade 3 invasive ductal carcinoma with medullary features.

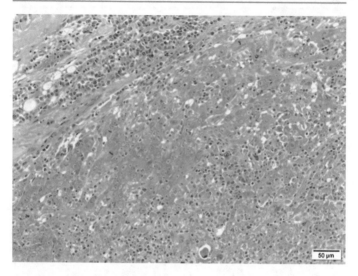

Fig. 5.38 Invasive medullary carcinoma

3. Metaplastic carcinomas

This is a group of breast carcinomas where the neoplastic cells acquire features that are not normally present in breast epithelium. Several varieties are described:

(a) <u>**Spindle cell carcinoma:**</u> This is the commonest type of metaplastic breast carcinoma and is also thought to be the most common spindle cell lesion of the breast. Hence, it is advised to stain any spindle cell lesion encountered in a breast core biopsy for cytokeratin to prove or exclude the possibility of a spindle cell carcinoma. The tumour cells acquire a sarcomatous spindle shape, but remain cytokeratin positive (Fig. 5.39). The degree of cellular differentiation is variable with some cases showing marked nuclear pleomorphism and others have a bland cytology that can be confused with benign fibromatosis, hence the name fibromatosis-like spindle cell carcinoma. Malignant glandular elements in the form of in situ or invasive ductal carcinoma may be present (Fig. 5.38a), but it should not

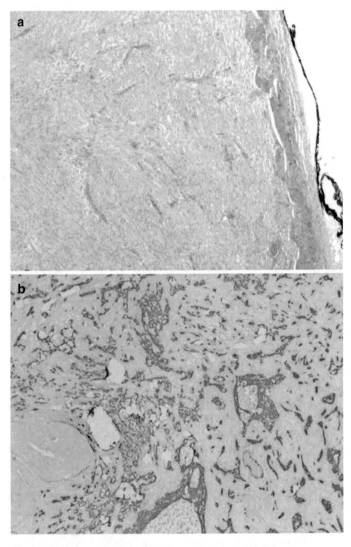

Fig. 5.39 Metaplastic spindle cell carcinoma: (**a**) H&E; (**b**) Pancytokeratin staining (AE1/AE3)

exceed 20% of the whole surface area of the sections examined to call the case pure metaplastic carcinoma. Squamous elements are not uncommonly seen mixed with the spindle cell elements (Fig. 5.40).

When testing for the presence of cytokeratin, at least two cytokeratin markers should be used as there is no single marker that can stain all spindle cell carcinomas. The two most commonly used, and most frequently expressed, markers are AE1/AE3 and MNF116, but other markers like CK8/18, CK19 or p63 can be also useful [49].

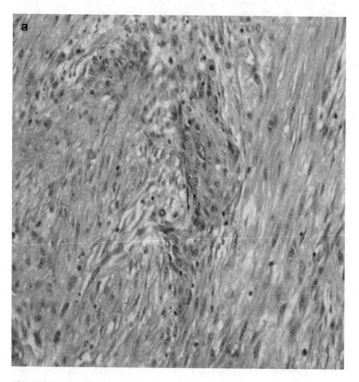

Fig. 5.40 Metaplastic mixed spindle cell/squamous carcinoma: (**a**) H&E; (**b**) Pan-cytokeratin

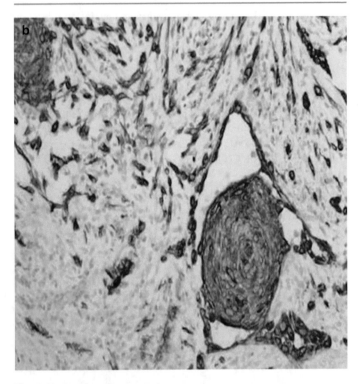

Fig. 5.40 (continued)

(b) **<u>Squamous cell carcinoma</u>:** Pure squamous cell carcinoma
of the breast is extremely rare (Fig. 5.41), and the possibility of the lesion being a direct extension from a skin squamous carcinoma or a metastasis from other organs, like
lung, cervix or oesophagus, should be excluded before
confirming a primary origin in the breast. Mixed spindle/
squamous carcinomas as described above (Fig. 5.40) are
more common than pure squamous carcinoma. I have also
seen a case of ER negative squamous cell carcinoma in
continuity with an ER positive invasive ductal carcinoma.

(c) **<u>Adeno-squamous carcinoma</u>:** <u>low and high grade</u>: This is
another variant of metaplastic carcinoma where the glandu-

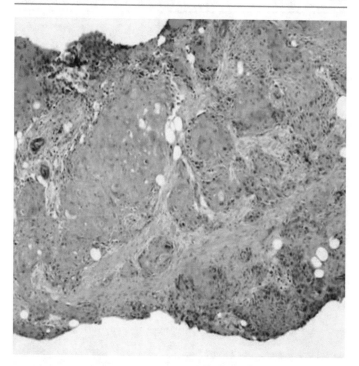

Fig. 5.41 Metaplastic squamous cell carcinoma, core biopsy

lar and squamous neoplastic elements are intimately mixed with each other. Microscopically, the low grade type consists of scattered low grade glandular and squamous elements, intimately associated or even linked in a markedly desmoplastic stroma, resembling a scar (Fig. 5.42). The prognosis is excellent [50]. On the other hand, in high grade adenosquamous carcinoma the two elements are of a high grade and the prognosis is poor (Fig. 5.43). Cytokeratins are positive in all elements and p63 is positive in the squamous areas (Fig. 5.43b, c).

(d) **Matrix producing carcinoma:**

This is defined as invasive breast carcinoma with a direct transition of carcinoma to myxochondroid matrix without an intervening spindle cell component [51–53].

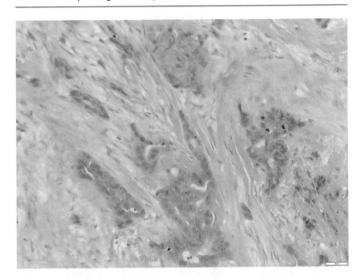

Fig. 5.42 Low grade adenosquamous carcinoma

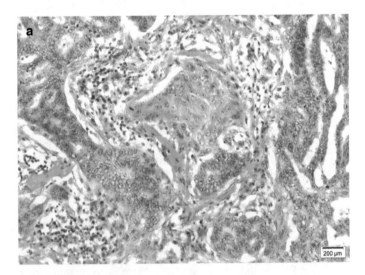

Fig. 5.43 High grade adenosquamous carcinoma: (**a**) H&E; (**b**) CK14; (**c**) p63

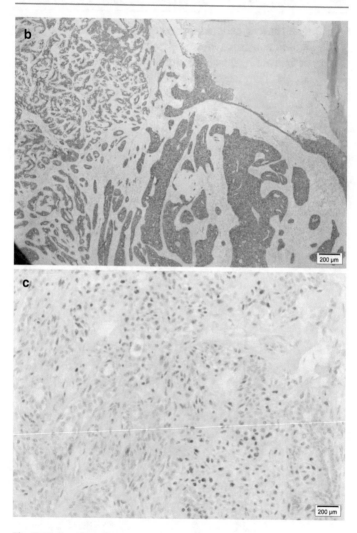

Fig. 5.43 (continued)

The tumour cells are arranged in nests, cords or sheets within a myxochondroid stroma (Fig. 5.44). The tumour cells usually show a moderate or high degree of nuclear atypia. They are positive for cytokeratin and negative for

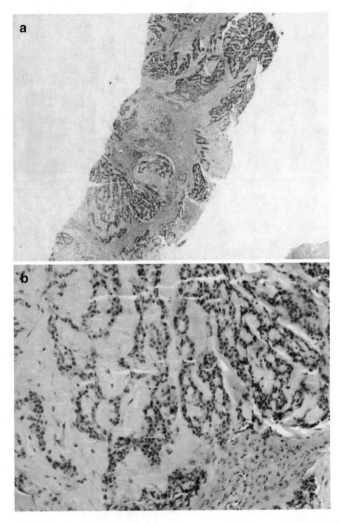

Fig. 5.44 Matrix producing metaplastic carcinoma, this case was associated with microglandular adenosis: (**a**) Low power view of a core biopsy; (**b**) high power view

ER, PR and HER2. They can be positive for p63. The matrix is positive for the cartilage specific matrix molecules aggrecan and type II collagen [52]. The ratio of matrix/cells varies from one case to another ranging from less than 10 to more than 40% [53]. Patients with tumours composed of more than 40% matrix tended to have a better distant-recurrence free survival, but the presence or absence of lympho-vascular invasion was more important in determining the prognosis, which is in general more aggressive than invasive ductal carcinoma [53]

(e) **Mixed metaplastic carcinoma:**

In addition to the common association of spindle cell and squamous elements in metaplastic breast carcinomas, other combinations, like spindle and metaplastic, do occur. An unusual metaplastic carcinoma seen in our department included matrix producing areas as well as squamous, spindle cell and in situ and invasive mucinous elements (Fig. 5.45).

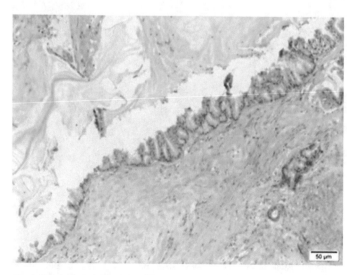

Fig. 5.45 Mucinous area seen in a metaplastic carcinoma

4. **Salivary gland-type carcinomas**

These are breast carcinomas that are more commonly seen in salivary glands. Four subtypes are known;

(a) **Adenoid cystic carcinoma:**

This is the commonest subtype of this group. The tumour cells are a mixture of epithelial and myoepithelial/basal cells arranged mostly in variable sized groups with a cribriform pattern (Fig. 5.46). Solid areas may be present and the tumours can be graded according to the amount of solid areas present into grade I, II and III, with more solid areas indicating a higher grade. Most tumours are grade I with no or little solid areas present and the prognosis of these is excellent [54]. Immunohistochemically, the tumours are triple negative and are positive for basal markers (Fig. 5.46d) and are mostly positive for CD117 (Fig. 5.46e) and show strong nuclear positivity for MYB [55].

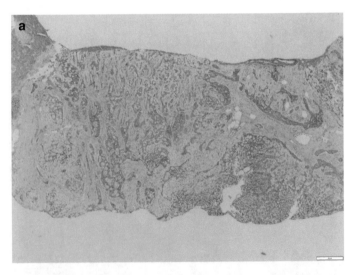

Fig. 5.46 Adenoid cystic carcinoma: (**a**) Low power view of a core biopsy; (**b**) high power view; (**c**) Negative ER staining; (**d**) positive CK5; (**e**) positive CD117

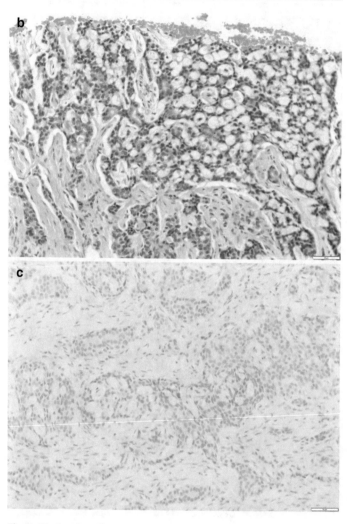

Fig. 5.46 (continued)

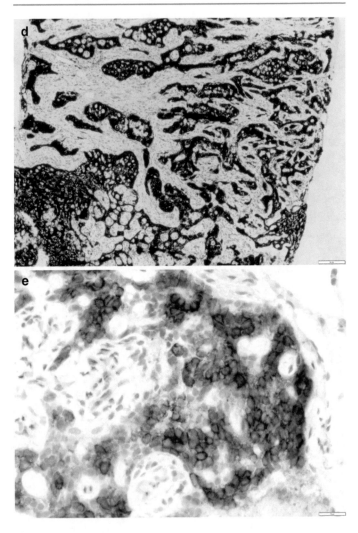

Fig. 5.46 (continued)

(b) Secretory carcinoma

This tumour is more common in younger patients, including children, although it can occur at any ages in both sexes. The tumours usually present as well defined sub-areolar mass. Microscopically, the cells have abundant granular eosinophilic cytoplasm and low grade nuclei [56]. The cells are arranged in glandular, cystic, microcystic, cribriform or solid pattern characterised by the presence of abundant extracellular and intracellular eosinophilc secretion that stains positively with PAS or Alcian Blue (Fig. 5.47). The tumours are triple negative, stain strongly positive for S100 (Fig. 5.47e) and the majority stain for basal markers like cytokeratin 5 and 14. Genomically, the tumour harbours the chromosomal translocation t(12;15) that results in a fusion of the ETS variant gene 6 (ETV6) on 12p13 and the neurotrophic tyrosine kinase receptor 3 (NTRK3) on 15q25. The prognosis is usually very good.

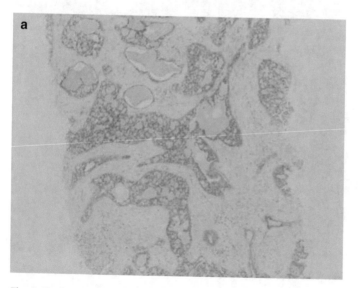

Fig. 5.47 Secretory carcinoma; (**a**) Low power view of a core biopsy; (**b**) High power view. (**c**) Further high power view showing the eosinophilic secretion; (**d**) Negative ER staining; (**e**) strong S100 positive staining

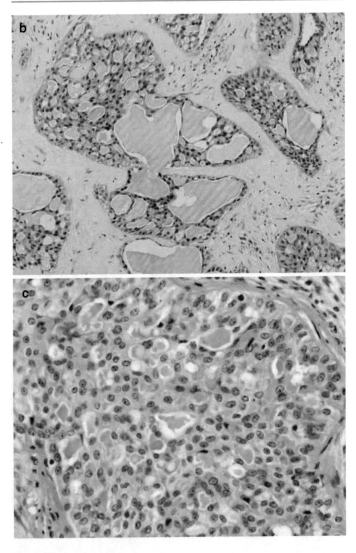

Fig. 5.47 (continued)

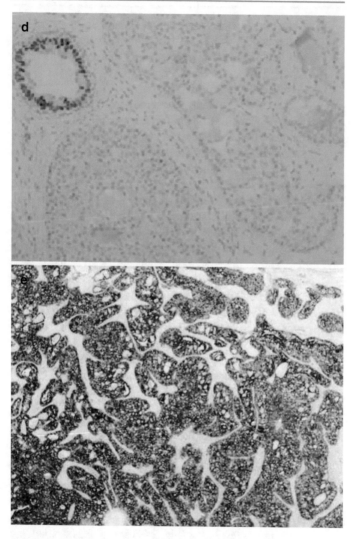

Fig. 5.47 (continued)

Lymph node metastases are uncommon, local recurrence, if developed, is late, distant metastasis are exceedingly rare and death from the disease is unusual but has been reported [56].

(c) **Acinic cell carcinoma**

This is an extremely rare tumour with microscopic features similar to those of secretory carcinoma where the tumour cells are arranged in glandular microcystic or solid structures but differ from the cells of secretory carcinoma by the presence of cytoplasmic coarse zymogen granules similar to the granules seen in Paneth cells (Fig. 5.48). The granules are positive for amylase, alpha-1-chymotrypsin, lysozyme, EMA, Diastase PAS and S100. They can also be positive for GCDFP-15. Cells with clear cytoplasm can be also present [57, 58]. The tumour is purely epithelial with no mixed myoepithelial elements. Cases have been described where acinic cell carcinoma was seen merging with microglandular adenosis and the two lesions may be related [59]. The tumour is described as having a low aggressive potential [58]. In 30 reported patients, axillary node metastasis were present in around 30%, distant metastasis in liver, bone and lung in around 10% and death in 6% after an average follow up of 42 months [58].

(d) **Epithelial myoepithelial carcinoma/malignant adeno-myoepithelioma**

This is another rare not well characterised invasive breast tumour composed of malignant glandular and myoepithelial elements. Some cases present in association with benign adenomyoepithelioma [60]. The ratio of the epithilial to myoepthelial elements varies from one case to another. The myoepithelial elements can be cuboidal or spindle shaped and can be present around the glandular structures as few layers (Fig. 5.49) or as sheets surrounding a few glandular structures (Fig. 5.50). The glandular structures may be simple or complex with papillary projections (Fig. 5.49a, b). The neoplastic cells usually show a moderate degree of nuclear pleomorphism. Areas of squamous differentiation, haemorrhage and necrosis may be present. Both elements are usually triple negative [61, 62]. The

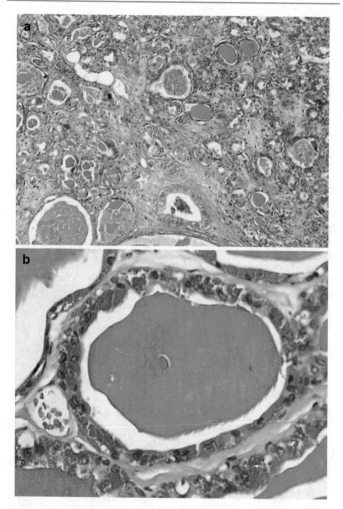

Fig. 5.48 Acinic cell carcinoma: (**a**) Low power view; (**b**) High power view showing the cytoplasmic zymogen granules

presence of myoepithelium around the glandular structures raises the possibility of a benign or in situ malignant lesion, but immunohistochemistry shows that both elements are triple negative and frankly invasive elements are commonly present at the periphery of the lesion (Fig. 5.50b).

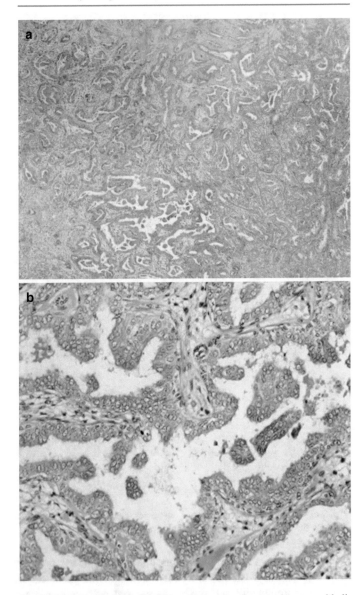

Fig. 5.49 Epithelial/myoepithelial carcinoma (malignant adenonyoepitheli-oma), well differentiated: (**a**) Low power view; (**b**) High power view; (**c**) p63 staining showing negative luminal and positive myoepithelial cells

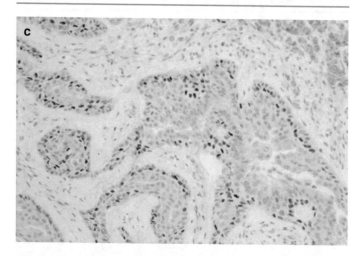

Fig. 5.49 (continued)

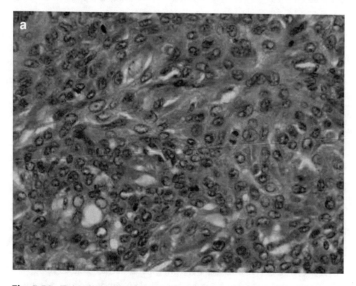

Fig. 5.50 Epithelial/myoepithelial carcinoma (malignant adenonyoepithelioma), poorly differentiated: (**a**) H&E; (**b**) CK5

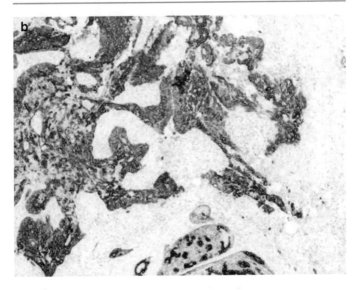

Fig. 5.50 (continued)

(e) **Malignant Myoepithelioma**

This is a rare triple negative malignant tumour composed entirely of myoepithelial cells which could be rounded, polyhedral or spindle shaped (Fig. 5.51). The cells are positive for myoepithelil/basal cell markers, e.g. cytokeratin 5 (Fig. 5.51b), p63, SMA and CD10. Cytokeratin 8/18 may be also positive (Fig. 5.51c). The tumour may arise de novo or in a pre-existing benign adenomyoepithelioma. In a study of 15 patients, all were female with an age range of 45–86 years, 14 presenting as a solid mass 10–48 mm, and one was cystic. Axillary lymph node metastasis and distal metastasis have been described, but the prognosis in general is favourable [63].

5. **Carcinoma associated with microglandular adenosis**

A variety of breast carcinomas have been described arising in association with micrglandular adenosis. They are all characterised, like microglandular adenosis itself, by being triple negative and S100 strongly positive (Fig. 5.52). In addition, there are

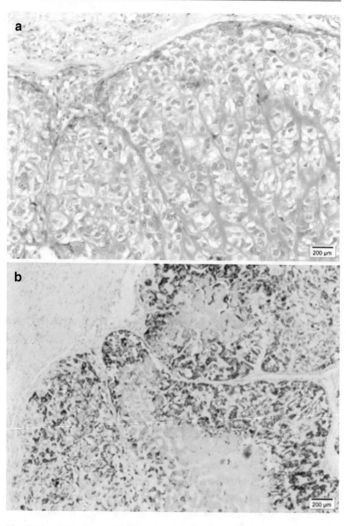

Fig. 5.51 Malignant myoepithelioma: (**a**) H&E; (**b**) CK5; (**c**) CK 8/18

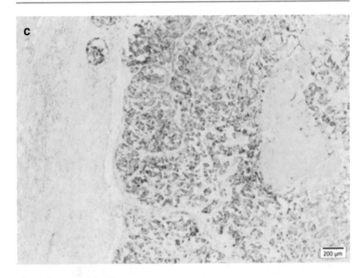

Fig. 5.51 (continued)

molecular similarities between the two lesions and it is not uncommon to find transitiobal foci of atypical microglandular adenosis leading to the invasive tumour (Fig. 5.52c). Cases reported include invasive ductal (Fig. 5.52), lobular, adenoid cystic, metaplastic (Fig. 5.44) and acinic cell carcinoma [59, 64].

Grading of Primary Invasive Breast Carcinoma

This is an essential part of reporting core biopsies. It is usually more accurate than grading the excised tumour because of the small size of the biopsy and its immediate insertion in formalin, thus guaranteeing good fixation. Also, many patients now have neo-adjuvant chemotherapy and the grade of the tumour is an important factor in deciding whether or not to administer such therapy. In addition, as chemotherapy might change the grade of the tumour or might cause its complete disappearance, grading the tumour in core biopsies preserves a record of its original actual grade.

For invasive carcinoma, the Elston and Ellis grading method is used which depends on the assessment of three histological features: the extent of glandular differentiation, the degree of nuclear pleomorphism and the number of mitotic figures [65]. A score of

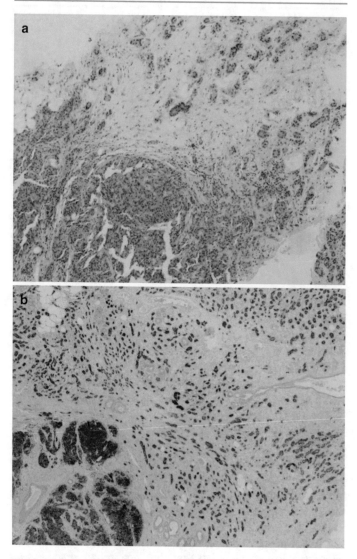

Fig. 5.52 Invasive ductal carcinoma arising in association with microglandular adenosis: (**a**) H&E; (**b**) S100 staining; (**c**) Atypical microglandular adenosis leading to the carcinoma

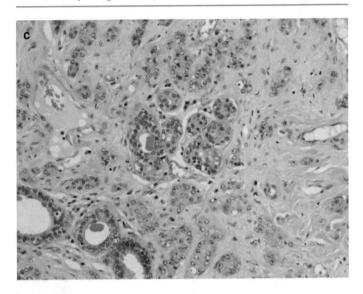

Fig. 5.52 (continued)

1–3 is assigned to each feature. The added total scores for the three features determine the tumour grade.

Thus, for glandular differentiation, a score of 1 is given if >75% of the tumour cells are arranged in glandular structures, a score of 2 if glands form 10–75% of the tumour, and a score of 3 is given if the glands are <10%.

Nuclear pleomorphism is assessed as for DCIS, with a score of 1 given to low grade nuclei, a score of 2 for intermediate grade, and a score of three for high grade nuclei. The low grade nuclei are uniform and near normal size which is 1.5–2.0 times the size of red blood cell or normal duct epithelial nucleus. The high grade nuclei are markedly pleomorphic with many being more than 2.5 times the size of RBC or normal duct epithelial nucleus. Intermediate grade nuclei show a moderate degree of nuclear pleomorphism which is less than that seen in high grade lesions but lacks the nuclear and cellular monotony of low grade lesions.

For mitotic activity, the score depends on the number of mitotic figures/10 high power microscopic fields (HPF), and the diameter of this field. For a field diameter of 0.48, a score of 1 is given for 0–6 mitoses/10 HPF, a score of 2 for 7–12 mitoses, and a score of 3 for >12 mitoses.

On adding the 3 scores together, a total score of 3–5 indicates a grade 1 tumour, a total score of 6–7 is a grade 2, and 8–9 indicates a greed 3 invasive tumour.

All carcinomas are graded regardless of their histological type, although the grade of certain histological types is always constant because of how they look like microscopically. For example, tubular carcinomas are always grade 1 as they have abundant glands, low or intermediate nuclei and low mitotic activity (Fig. 5.26); invasive lobular carcinoma, classical type is mostly grade 2 as glandular formation is uncommon and nuclear pleomorphism and mitotic activity are low or intermediate (Fig. 5.18) while medullary and medullary like carcinomas are always grade 3 because of the absence of glandular differentiation, marked nuclear pleomorphism and high mitotic count (Fig. 5.38).

Other Additional Features That Should Be Mentioned in the Core Biopsy Report

(a) **The presence or absence of DCIS:** The presence of abundant DCIS elements in association with an invasive carcinoma in a core biopsy, may be an indication that the whole tumour has an extensive DCIS component [66]. This is thought by some authors to be a risk factor for positive lumpectomy margin status, particularly for DCIS, which might necessitates wider than usual local excision [66]. Thus a comment on the extent of DCIS elements in relation to the invasive tumour, may have practical implications.

(b) **Calcification:** It is important to state in the report whether microcalcification is present or not and if present whether it is associated with the invasive tumour or with foci of DCIS or benign change like columnar cell change or flat epithelial atypia that may also be present in the biopsy. This is particularly important if the biopsy was done for radiological microcalcification and a decision has to be made about the extent of the surgical excision.

(c) **Necrosis:** In invasive carcinomas, necrosis is more commonly seen in high grade tumours, particularly triple negative ones. If seen in a core biopsy, it is worth mentioning in the report as its presence is thought to be one of the factors associated with a higher incidence of complete pathological response after neo-adjuvant chemotherapy [67].

(d) **Elastosis:** This is more common in low grade carcinomas and its presence is thought to be associated with good prognosis. Elastosis is not usually seen in extra-mammary carcinomas metastasising to the breast, which can be a useful feature to differentiate primary from metastatic carcinoma in the breast.

(e) **Lymphocytic infiltration (Tumour infiltrating lymphocytes; TILs)**

Assessing the extent of lymphocytic infiltration in the stroma of the tumour in a core biopsy is particularly useful in triple negative and HER2 positive tumours as it has been shown to have a prognostic significance. In triple negative tumours, high lymphocytic count was shown to be associated with lower recurrence [68], with each 10% increase in the count producing better survival [69]. Similar effect was seen in HER2 positive tumours [68, 70]. Increased concentrations of TILs was also shown to be a predictor of response to neo-adjuvant chemotherapy with complete pathological response noted in $$% of tumours with high concentration of TILS compared with 22% of tumours with low TILs [71] and it is thought that a high lymphocytic count reflects a favourable [71] host anti-tumour response [70].

Following are the recommendations of an International TILs working group on how to evaluate tumour infiltrating lymphocytes [72]:

- TILs should be reported for the stromal component as a percentage of the area occupied by lymphocytes (and plasma cells, but not neutrophils) over the total stromal area within the borders of the invasive tumour
- Exclude lymphocytes outside tumour, overlying the tumour, around DCIS, and in necrotic areas
- One representative section of the tumour is enough, the whole section is analysed, not a hot spot
- An example: 80% TILS means that 80% of the stromal area shows dense mononuclear infiltrate.
- The Committee did not recommend any relevant threshold for clinical use

Example of triple negative tumours with 0, 30 and 90% TILs are illustrated in Fig. 5.53. Tumours with more lymphocytes than tumour cells (Fig. 5.53c) are sometimes called lymphocytes-predominant breast cancer or lympho-epithelioma-like carcinoma.

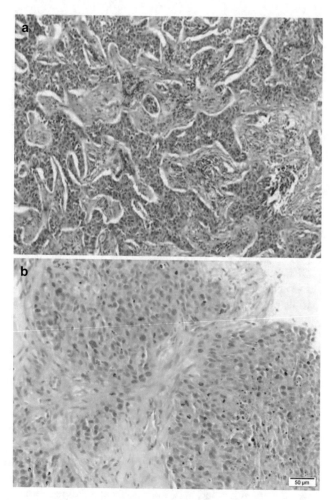

Fig. 5.53 Triple negative invasive ductal carcinoma with: (**a**) around 30% tumour infiltrating lymphocytes (TILs), (**b**) 0% TILS; (**c**) 90%

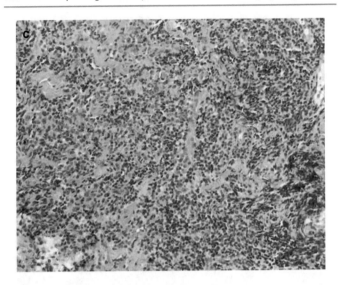

Fig. 5.53   (continued)

High concentrations of TILs, defined as 60% or more, have been detected in 30% of triple negative tumours compared with 19% of HER2 positive and 13% of ER positive, HER2 negative tumours [71]. Complete pathological response following neo-adjuvant chemotherapy was noted in 50% of triple negative tumours with high TILs concentration and in 48% of HER2 positive tumours and in 28% of ER positive, HER2 negative tumours with high TILs count [71].

On the other hand, it is common to see lymphocytic aggregates at the edge of invasive lobular carcinoma. This sometimes helps in confirming the lobular phenotype of the tumour, although the significance of these aggregates is not known.

(f) **lympho-vascular invasion:** The presence of lympho-vascular invasion should not be stated in a core biopsy report unless there is no doubt whatsoever that this is the case, as shrinkage artefacts can mimic lymphatic invasion. The presence of the suspected focus outside the tumour and particularly if it is associated with adjacent blood vessels, can help differentiating real vascular invasion from shrinkage artefacts.

(g) **Receptor and HER2 status:** Assessment of ER, PR and HER2 status of invasive carcinoma using immunohistochemistry is an essential part of a core biopsy report. However, as these are not usually requested until a diagnosis of invasive carcinoma is made, an immediate report is usually issued including all the information discussed above, with a supplementary report issued later, usually within a day or two, containing the immunohistochemical results of the receptors and HER2 assessments.

ER and PR Assessment

This assessment is now routinely done immunohistochemically using the immunoperoxidase technique and routinely processed paraffin sections of the tumour. Highly specific monoclonal antibodies that work in paraffin sections are commercially available.

- Using specific antibodies, positive staining is identified as dark brown nuclear staining of the tumour cells (Fig. 5.54). Proper positive and negative controls should be used in each batch of

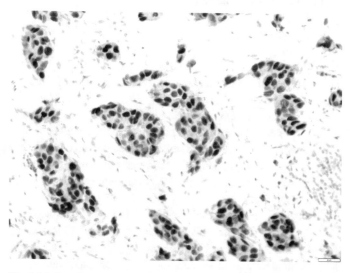

Fig. 5.54 Invasive ductal carcinoma with an Allred score of 8/8, H. score 300

staining. Only nuclear staining of tumour cells is taken into consideration, any cytoplasmic staining, which is occasionally seen, is ignored as it is thought to be non-specific.

- The results are usually scored semi-quantitatively for routine use, although quantitative methods are also available.
- There are two different ways of scoring the results both relying on the percentage of stained cells and the intensity of the stain. Allred Score [73] is currently the most commonly used scoring system. The score is arrived at by adding 2 numbers:
- One number reflecting the % of positively stained cells (this is carried out by scanning the stained section by the low power and estimating the % of positive cells):
  - 0 none
  - 1 for <1%
  - 2 for 1–10%
  - 3 for 11–33%
  - 4 for 34–66%
  - 5 for >67%
- And the other number reflecting the intensity of staining (of the majority of stained cells):
  - 1 weak,
  - 2 moderate
  - 3 strong
- Resulting in a scale of 0/8 to 8/8
  - A score of 0/8 (All tumour cells are negative) + Negative

    Three is no score of 1/8,

    A score of 2/8 (indicating less than 1% of tumour cells are weakly stained) is considered to be negative.

    A score of 3/8 would be considered negative if less than 1% of tumour cells show moderate staining (1 + 2), and weakly positive if 1–10% of tumour cells show weak staining (2 + 1)

    A score of 4/8 would be considered negative if less than 1% of tumour cells are strongly positive (1 + 3), and weakly positive if more than 1% of tumour cells show moderate positive staining (2 + 2) or larger number of cells show weak staining (3 + 1)

A score of 5/8 also indicates weak positivity

A score of 6/8 indicates moderate positivity

Scores of 7/8 and 8/8 usually considered to indicate a strong positivity

It has to be mentioned here that some authorities require at least 10% of the tumour cells to be positively stained to consider the case as ER positive, while others have observed positive response to anti-oestrogen therapy in the presence of only one positive tumour cell in the section examined.

- The other scoring system (the H score) uses the same principle of the Allred score by giving the weak staining a score of 1, moderate a score of 2 and strong staining a score of 3. Then multiplying the intensity score with the actual percentage of the positively stained cells. Thus, if all the tumour cells are strongly stained, the resulting H score is 300 (3×100). A score of more than 200 is considered strong and is given +++. A score 200–300 is moderate, ++, 50 or more is weakly positive (1+) and less than 50 is negative. The Allred and H scores can be converted to each other if needed, for example when comparing results of treatment from centres using one or the other scoring system [74]

- Giving this type of semi-quantitative result is useful, as there are indications that the higher the score the more likely that the patient will respond to hormonal treatment.

- Staining and scoring should be carried out according to a strict protocol, and ideally the laboratory should participate in a National or Regional Quality Assurance Schemes to guarantee the quality of the procedure.

- Assessment of ER is more commonly done than PR (progesterone receptors), but the latter can be useful in the rare cases which are ER negative, PR positive, as some of these patients may respond to hormone treatment. Also, there are indications that the response rate of ER and PR positive tumours is higher than ER positive, PR negative ones. Lastly PR status is included in the new Pathologic prognostic staging system

- The same scoring systems can be used for assessing the receptor status of DCIS if needed, for example to decide if the patient can be offered Tamoxifen as an adjuvant therapy or not.

HER2 Assessment [75]

Assessment of HER2 receptor status is recommended for all primary breast carcinomas in order to decide whether the patient will need anti-HER2 therapy or not. This is best carried out on the original core biopsy used for making the diagnosis. The test can be done on a fine needle aspirate if this is the only material available for the primary diagnosis, or on excised tumour tissue, if the test was not done before surgery or if it was done but the result is not available. The test is also recommended for all recurrent and metastatic carcinomas from which tissue samples are available.

- The specimen to be tested should have been put in 10% neutral buffered formalin within 1 h of removal from the breast and left to fix for 6–72 h. If the test was carried out on a core biopsy, there is no need to repeat it on the excised tumour except in the following situations:
    - The test was HER2 positive in an ER/PR positive grade 1 invasive ductal carcinoma or in pure tubular, cribriform, mucinous or adenoid cystic carcinoma.
    - Additional tumours of different morphology were found in the excised specimen
    - The original result on the core was equivocal even after in situ hybridization (ISH) testing.
- The tumour should be first tested by immunohistochemistry (IHC) and the results interpreted as follows:
    - − (negative): No membrane staining or faint, incomplete membrane staining in 10% or less of invasive tumour cells
    - + (negative): Faint incomplete membrane staining in more than 10% of invasive tumour cells
    - ++ (equivocal): Weak to moderate complete membrane staining in more than 10% of invasive tumour cells, or strong complete membrane staining in 10% or less. Proceed with in situ hybridisation (ISH, see below).
    - +++ (positive): Intense dark contiguous, homogenous, complete membrane staining (chicken wire pattern) in more than 10% of invasive tumour cells (Fig. 5.55).

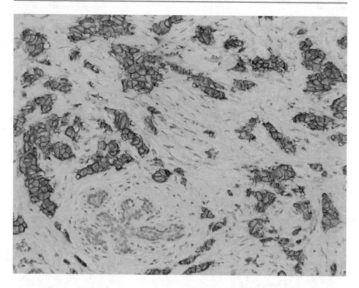

Fig. 5.55 Invasive ductal carcinoma with HER2 immunohistochemistry sore of +++

- For multiple tumours:
  - If all foci are of the same histological type and grade: Assess only the largest focus.
  - Do additional assessment for any focus with a different histology or grade
- In situ hybridisation should be carried out for all cases scoring ++ (equivocal) with IHC, to determine if there is meaningful amplification of the HER2 gene:
- Two techniques are currently available for detection of HER2 gene copy number using specific HER2 DNA probes
  - FISH (Fluorescent in situ hybridisation)
  - SISH (Silver enhanced in situ hybridisation)
- In both techniques, either a single probe for HER2 is used (to get a HER2 copy number), or dual colour probes are used, one for HER2 and the other for centromere 17 (CEP17). The latter is used as a reference probe reflecting the copy number of chromosome 17 where the HER2 gene is also located.

- If a dual colour probes are used the result is given as HER2/CEP 17 ratio (Fig. 5.56). If the test is done with a single probe for HER2, a parallel section can be used for assessing Chromosome 17 to get the HER2/CEP17 ratio.

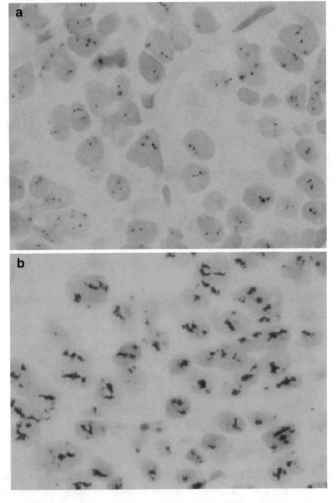

Fig. 5.56 Invasive ductal carcinoma: (**a**) HER2 SISH negative: The HER2 (black)/CEP 17 (red) ratio is less than 2. (**b**) HER2 SISH positive: HER2/CEP 17 ratio is more than 4

- All methods use routine paraffin sections and give comparable results [76]. SISH has the advantage of using ordinary light microscopes.
- Interpretation of ISH results:

  The signals obtained by the staining are counted in 20 cells and the average number of signals per cells is calculated.

  - The following indicate a positive HER2 result:

    Single probe: average HER2 copy number 6 signals or more/cell.

    Dual probe: An average HER2 copy number of 6 or more if the HER2/CEP17 ratio is less than 2, but only an average HER2 copy number of 4 or more if the HER2/CEP17 ratio is 2 or more

  - The following indicate an equivocal HER2 result:

    Single probe: average HER2 copy number 4–6 signals/cell.

    Dual probe: HER2 copy number 4–6 signals/cell and a HER2/CEP17 ratio less than 2

  - The following indicate a negative HER2 result:

    Single probe: average HER2 copy number less than 4 signals/cell.

    Dual probe: An average HER2 copy number less than 4 signals/cell whatever the HER2/CEP ratio is

    Dual probe: An average HER2 copy number of 4 or more but less than 6 signals/cell and HER2/CEP ratio is less than 2

  - To summarise, a case is considered HER2 ISH positive if there is an average HER2 copy number of 6 signals or more/cell. However, if dual probes are used and the HER2/CEP ratio is 2 or more, an average of 4 HER2 copy numbers is enough to consider the case positive.

  - In equivocal cases the signals are counted in more cells (20 at a time) until a conclusion is reached.

  - Cases that stay equivocal after repeated counting (and are originally equivocal by IHC) have been labelled as HER2 double equivocal and found to be mostly Luminal B and show high risk of recurrence [77].

- The result should be considered indeterminate If technical issues prevent accurate interpretation, either because of inadequate specimen handling or because of the presence of artefacts, like crushing, which hinders assessment.

Other Immunohistological Studies

Sometimes, other immunostains may have to used to establish or confirm a diagnosis. For example Cytokeratin, for confirming the presence of small foci of metastasis in a lymph node or establishing the diagnosis of metaplastic carcinoma in spindle cell lesions; E-Cadherin, to differentiate between lobular and ductal lesions in questionable cases; myoepithelial markers, e.g. p63, smooth muscle actin or CD10, to confirm the diagnosis of tubular carcinoma (no myoepithelial cells) or differentiate between in situ and invasive carcinoma in questionable cases and Gross Cystic Disease Fluid Protein (GCDFP)-15 to confirm the diagnosis of apocrine carcinoma (strong diffuse positive staining).

Molecular Classification of Breast Carcinoma

This classification can usually be deduced once the hormone receptors and HER2 status of the tumour is known. There are four main molecular types as follows:

1. Luminal A:
   (a) ER positive
   (b) PR positive (more than 20%)
   (c) HER2 negative
   (d) These tumours usually have a low Ki67 score (less than 20%) and low Oncotype DXRecurrence risk score. The tumours are usually low grade and have an excellent prognosis.
2. Luminal B
   (a) ER positive
   (b) HER2 can be negative or positive
      • HER2 negative
         – PR negative or low (less than 20%)
         – Ki67 high (more than 20%)
         – Oncotype DX recurrence risk high (more than 31)

- HER2 positive group:
  - PR any
  - Ki67 any
  (c) The tumours in both groups are usually high grade with poor prognosis.
3. HER2 positive group (which could be ER positive or negative). Tumours are usually high grade with poor prognosis
4. Basal like group
   (a) ER negative
   (b) PR negative
   (c) HER2 negative
   (d) Tumours are positive for at least one of the basal markers like CK5 or 14

The question usually arises: do we have to mention the molecular type in our reports? I do not think this is essential as it is not going to affect the management of the disease. More important is to mention the receptors and HER 2 status of the tumours are these are the main factors that affect the management.

Complete Removal of Lesions

With the introduction of wider needles for core biopsies, lesions may be removed in their entirety by this procedure. Thus, in a study of 51 cases of invasive carcinomas using stereotactic 11-gauge directional vacuum-assisted biopsy followed by surgical excision, no residual carcinoma was detected in 10 cases (20%). Complete excision was more likely to occur if 14 cores or more were taken [78]. In these cases, tumour size can be assessed either from the imaging studies done before the biopsy, or by measuring the tumour microscopically in the core biopsy. The latter measurement tends to underestimate the maximum dimension of the tumour [78]. For this reason, it is usually useful, when dealing with small lesions, to place a localising device, like a metal clip at the site of the biopsy after taking the cores, to facilitate accurate localisation of the lesion's site if subsequent surgical excision is expected to be carried out [79].

Primary Sarcomas of the Breast

These will be identified in a core biopsy as a highly cellular spindle cell lesion composed of closely packed interlacing or haphazardly arranged bundles of plump spindle shaped cells with prominent nuclear pleomorphism and mitotic activity (Fig. 5.57). Before making a diagnosis of sarcoma two other possibilities should be considered: malignant phyllodes tumour and metaplastic spindle cell carcinoma. The presence of scattered benign-looking glandular elements would indicate a malignant phyllodes tumour (Fig. 5.58). However, these epithelial elements may be scanty, hence multiple levels should be examined, or totally absent in recurrent tumours, but a history of a previous phyllodes in the same area should be enough to consider the lesion, in a core biopsy, as a recurrent phyllodes. The possibility of a metaplastic spindle cell carcinoma has to be always considered in spindle cell lesions of the breast by staining the sections by staining the sections for at least two epithelial markers. The two more commonly used are Ae1/AE3 and MNF116.

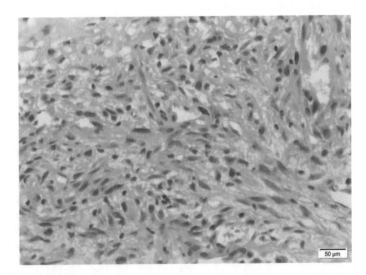

Fig. 5.57 High grade sarcoma composed of haphazardly arranged plump spindle shaped cells with prominent nuclear pleomorphosm and mitotic activity. No glandular elements are present and epithelial markers were negative

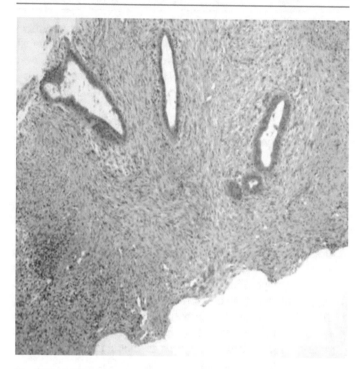

Fig. 5.58 Malignant phyllodes tumour: highly cellular spindle cell lesion with high nuclear pleomorphism and mitotic activity with scattered benign glandular elements

Once the possibilities of phyllodes tumour and spindle cell carcinoma, which are the most common malignant spindle cell lesions of the breast, have been excluded, other immunostains should be used to try to identify the cells' phenotype. That would include smooth muscle actin, desmin, S100, CD34, CD10 and possibly others, as primary sarcomas of all types have been described in the breast. These include leiomyosarcoma, rhabdomyosarcoma, fibrosarcoma, stromal sarcoma, liposarcoma, osteosarcoma, chondrosarcoma, angiosarcoma and giant cell tumour of soft tissue. In this respect it has to be remembered that rare tumours of the chest wall can present as breast lumps and we have seen two such cases one was an osteosarcoma and the other a giant cell tumour of soft tissue both arising in the chest wall and presenting clinically as breast lumps [80].

A variety of sarcomas in the breast can develop as a result of radiotherapy given as an adjuvant therapy for breast carcinoma. Perhaps the commonest is angiosarcoma, but other tumours have been described including fibrosarcoma and osteosarcoma.

Angiosarcoma

This is rare, but is the most common palpable vascular tumour of the breast, amounting to 62% of a large series of a 100 vascular tumours [81]

- It can arise either de novo, or, more commonly nowadays several years after therapeutic irradiation of the breast.
- Primary angiosarcoma usually occurs in younger women and often involves the breast parenchyma. Secondary angiosarcoma occurs in elderly women with history of breast cancer and irradiation, and is mostly cutaneous and multifocal[2]. The latter are responsible for the recent increase in the incidence of angiosarcoma of the breast [82]
- A study of 21 cases from the Netherlands has estimated the incidence of post-irradiation breast angiosarcoma as 0.16%, with a median interval between carcinoma and sarcoma of around 6 years and a range of 3–9 years [83].
- In post-irradiation angiosarcoma, the tumour arises either in the skin or in the breast tissue within the field of irradiation, and the main differential diagnosis is a recurrent carcinoma. Clinically, there are usually multiple bluish or purple skin nodules, purple skin discolourations, erythematous macules or areas, sometimes combined with ulceration, oedema or a palpable mass [84].
- The lesions are usually larger than 2 cm, ill-defined, soft and haemorrhagic.
- Microscopically, there are anastomosing vascular channels lined by atypical endothelial cells with hyperchromatic nuclei, as well as a variable amount of variable sized clumps of spindle-shaped cells. Areas of haemorrhage and necrosis may be present (Fig. 5.59).
- The diagnosis can be confirmed by immunoperoxidase stains for keratin and endothelial cells. A keratin stain would show only a few scattered positively stained benign mammary

glands, while the neoplastic cells being negative. An endothelial marker, e.g., CD31 and CD34, would positively stain at least some of the neoplastic endothelial cells.

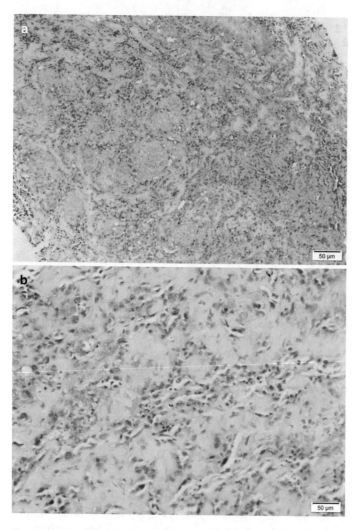

Fig. 5.59 Post-irradiation angiosarcoma, breast skin punch biopsy: (**a**) H&E, (**b**) High power view, (**c**) CD31 positive immunostaining

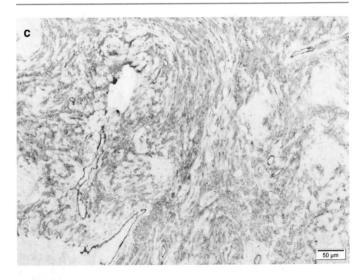

Fig. 5.59 (continued)

- Angiosarcoma of the breast has been classified into three grades which proved to be of prognostic significance. In grade III, there is endothelial tufting, papillary formation, solid and spindle cell areas and abundant mitoses. These features are absent or minimal in grade I, and are present only focally in grade II. In addition, grade III shows blood lakes and areas of necrosis. In a series of 63 cases, diagnosed mostly before 1981, the estimated 5-year disease-free survival was 76% for grade I, 70% for grade II and 15% for grade III; while the 5-year estimated survival probabilities were 91%, 68% and 14% respectively [85]. Most post-irradiation angiosarcomas are high grade and have a poor prognosis [84, 86, 87].
- Not all post-irradiation vascular lesions of the breast are malignant. Fineberg and Rosen have described a benign atypical vascular lesion developing in the breast or chest wall after post-operative irradiation [86]. These usually consist of dilated anastomosing irregular, usually empty, vascular channels lined by one or at most two layers of flat endothelial cells with plump hyperchromatic nuclei without nucleoli or obvious mitotic activity. The lumina of some of the channels may show

endothelium-lined stromal projections or septa. Lymphocytic infiltration and fibrosis are usually seen around the lesions. MYC gene amplification and protein expression are usually positive in post-irradiation angiosarcoma and negative in primary angiosarcoma and post-irradiation atypical vascular lesions of the breast skin [88].

- In a report of 49 cases of primary angiosarcoma of the breast with no history of previous irradiation, there was no relationship between grade and prognosis. In that series, the median recurrence-free and overall survival rates for all cases were 2.8 and 5.7 years respectively. This indicated that it is similar in behaviour to angiosarcoma of the skin and soft tissue, carrying a moderate risk of local recurrence and a high risk of metastasis and death [89]. However, a further report of 11 cases, mostly developing after radiotherapy, confirmed the presence of a relationship between grade and prognosis with local recurrence [84] and distant metastases occurring only in high grade tumours [90].
- Angiosarcoma has been reported in a long standing (28 years) silicone implant capsule, with extensive lung metastasis and no history of previous breast carcinoma or radiotherapy [91].

Mammary Sarcoma with CD10 Expression
(Fig. 5.**60**)

- A breast sarcoma characterized by strong CD10 expression.
- In a report of seven cases [92], in addition to CD10 and vimentin positivity, there was EGFR expression in five, SMA and CD29 in three cases and p63 and calponin in two cases each. All seven tumours were negative for CK5/6, 34BE12, CK14, CK17, ER, PgR, CD34, desmin and h-caldesmon.
- According to that report, the absence of CD34 expression differentiates these tumours from other sarcomas including malignant phyllodes tumour and stromal sarcoma.
- The authors suggested that CD10 expression in these tumours indicates that these are sarcomas 'with myoepithelial features'. The prognosis was not discussed.

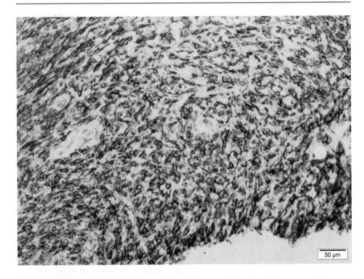

Fig. 5.60 CD10 positive high grade sarcoma of the breast

Stromal Sarcoma
- This term should be restricted to the rare examples of breast sarcomas which show unequivocal evidence of origin from specialised, lobular, mammary stroma. This can be confirmed by the presence of prominent stromal proliferation in intact lobules adjacent to the tumour [93].
- Probably equivalent to malignant phyllodes tumour, but with the absence of epithelial elements.

Primary Osteogenic Sarcoma
- This is one of the rarest tumours. One (3%) out of 32, and three (5%) out of 60 breast sarcomas reported by Callery et al. [93] and Gutman et al. [94] respectively were osteogenic sarcomas
- A major reference centre in the United States, The Armed Forces Institute of Pathology, Washington, DC, collected only 50 cases in around 40 years [95].
- These 50 cases included 49 women and 1 man, with age range of 27–89 years (median 64).
- 70% of the patients had symptoms for less than 2 months, 6% had a recent history of trauma and 4% had previous radiotherapy

- Tumour size varied between 1.4 and 13 cm (mean 4.6).
- Histology was fibroblastic in 56% (5 year survival 67%), osteoclastic in 28% and osteoblastic in 16% (5 year survival 31%). Stains for keratin, ER and PgR were always negative.
- Axillary lymph node dissection was carried out in 20 patients and all were free of tumour.
- Follow up information was available for 39 patients: 28% had local recurrence (mean 10 months) and 38% had distal metastases, most commonly in the lung (mean 14 months). The 5-year survival rate was 38%. Prognosis was worst in patients with tumours larger than 4.6 cm.
- An increasing number of post-irradiation osteogenic sarcomas are being reported, usually several years after therapeutic irradiation for breast carcinoma [96]. Most of these cases, however, arise from the chest wall and related bones rather than within residual breast tissue.

Lymphoma (Fig. 5.61)

- Lymphomas of the breast are rare, accounting for less than 0.5% of breast neoplasms [97].
- They can arise as a primary tumour of the breast, or involve the breast in a setting of disseminated lymphoma. In two relatively large series of 45 and 22 cases, around 50% were primary and 50% secondary [98, 99]. In another series of 31 cases, only around one third of the cases were primary [100]. There are no morphological differences between primary and secondary cases [101].
- They are more commonly seen on the right side, usually presenting as a unilateral breast mass in a middle-aged woman, with features identical to those of a carcinoma [97, 102]. However, bilateral cases, primary or secondary, are not uncommon [101].
- There seems to be a distinct subgroup of aggressive lymphoma affecting young women which is frequently bilateral and often associated with current or recent pregnancy and is of Burkitt type [101, 102].
- The majority are B cell lymphomas, mostly of diffuse large B cell type [94, 96], but other types have been described including MALT [97, 99, 100], Burkitt-like lymphomas [97],

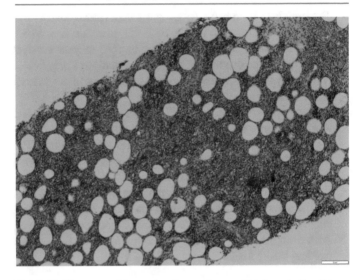

Fig. 5.61 Breast core biopsy showing a primary of high grade B cell lymphoma. H&E

Follicle-centre lymphoma [97, 99, 103], marginal zone lymphoma [103], lymphoplasmacytoid lymphoma [99], anaplastic large cell lymphoma [104] as well as a few well characterized cases of T-cell lymphomas [105, 106]. There are also reports of a few cases of Hodgkin's disease, nodular sclerosing type, involving the breast and chest wall and probably representing extra-nodal extension of the disease from intramammary, internal mammary or mediastinal lymph nodes [107].

- Lympho-epithelial lesions are identified in around two thirds of cases [101].
- Rare cases of primary breast lymphoma arising in postmastectomy lymphedema of the soft tissues of the arm 11–30 years after mastectomy, have been described [108].
- Treatment is usually by local radiotherapy which may be combined by the appropriate chemotherapy [97, 109].
- The prognosis of primary breast lymphoma is similar to that of nodal lymphomas of similar histological type and stage. In a series of 35 cases, the 5-year overall survival was 45% [110].

- More recently, a 'breast implant associated anaplastic large cell lymphoma' has been described arising in the capsule of breast implants of long standing [111]. The condition is rare and has a favourable prognosis

Metastatic Carcinoma in the Breast

Metastatic tumours to the breast from malignancy of other organs are not common, but should be always kept in mind when dealing with malignant breast core biopsies particularly when:

- On H&E the tumour has an unusual morphology that does not look like usual breast carcinomas like ductal, lobular, tubular, mucinous etc.
- A glandular malignant tumour that turned out, on immunohistochemistry, to be ER negative.
- The absence of in situ malignant elements or elastosis.

In such situations immunohistochemistry has to be carried out to confirm a non-mammary origin and to try to establish a possible primary origin. The list of antibodies used should be selected according to the morphology of the lesion. Useful antibodies include CK7, CK20, CDX2, GATA3, TTF1, WT1, CA125, CA19.9, S100 and HMB45. In a study of 85 cases of metastasis to the breast and axillary nodes in 72 female and 13 male, the primary tumour was melanoma in 22%, carcinoma in 49% and sarcomas in 18% [112]. The commonest primary carcinomas were in the ovary and lung with a few cases from the endometrium, colon, thyroid, pancreas, urinary bladder, kidney. Skin, prostate, tongue, choriocarcinoma and submandibular salivary glands. The commonest metastatic sarcoma with leiomyosarcoma with a few others including rhabdosarcoma, liposarcoma, malignant fibrous histiocytoma and synovial srcoma [112].

The morphology of the metastasis sometimes gives a clue to the most likely primary site, for example metastatic ovarian papillary adenocarcinoma with psammoma bodies, or metastatic colorectal carcinoma with wide areas of necrosis and negative ER expression (Fig. 5.62), or a metastaic clear renal cell carcinoma with negative ER and positive RCC expression (Fig. 5.63) or a metastatic leiomyosarcoma with closely packed malignant spindle cells which are positive for SMA and desmin (Fig. 5.64).

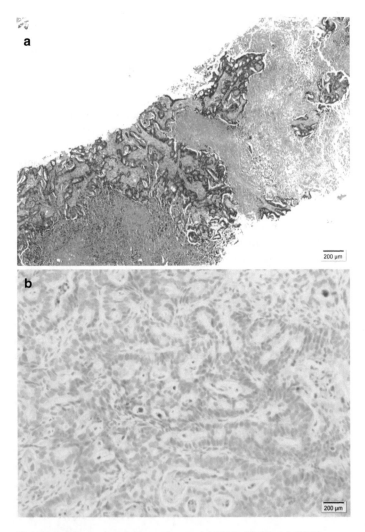

Fig. 5.62 Metastatic colonic carcinoma; (**a**) H&E, (**b**) ER, (**c**) CDX2

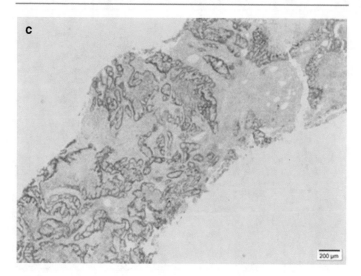

Fig. 5.62 (continued)

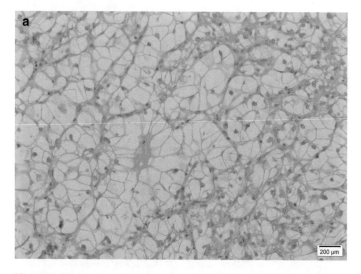

Fig. 5.63 Metastatic renal cell carcinoma: (**a**) H&E, (**b**) RCC immunohisto-chemistry

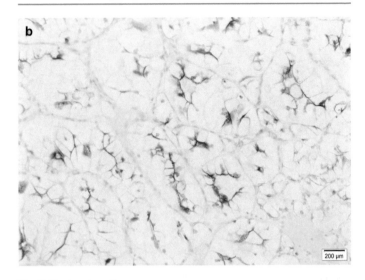

Fig. 5.63 (continued)

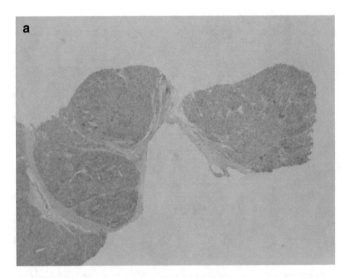

Fig. 5.64 Metastatic leiomyosarcoma, breast core biopsy (patient had uterine leiomyosarcoma) (**a**) H&E, (**b**) Desmin immunostaining

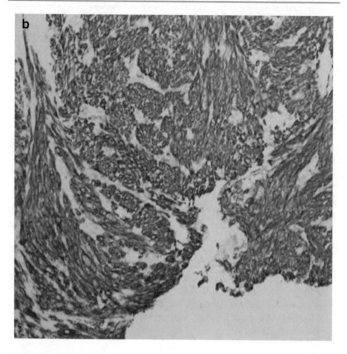

Fig. 5.64 (continued)

References

1. Shousha S, Forbes G, Hopkins I, Wright G. CD10 positive myoepithelial cells are usually prominent around in situ lobular neoplasia of the breast and much less prominent or absent in DCIS. J Clin Pathol. 2016;69(7): 702–5.
2. Baqai T, Shousha S. Oestrogen receptor negativity as a marker for high-grade ductal carcinoma in situ of the breast. Histopathology. 2003;42: 440–7.
3. Narod SA, Iqbal J, Giannakeas V, et al. Breast cancer mortality after a diagnosis of ductal carcinoma in situ. JAMA Oncol. 2015;1:888–96.
4. Roses RE, Arun BK, Lari SA, et al. Ductal carcinoma-in-situ of the breast with subsequent distant metastasis and death. Ann Surg Oncol. 2011;18:2873–8.

5. Visser LL, Elshof LE, Schaapveld M, et al. Clinicopathological risk factors for an invasive breast cancer recurrence after ductal carcinoma *in situ*—a nested case control study. Clin Cancer Res. 2018;24:3593–601.

6. Savage JL, Jeffries DO, Noroozian M, et al. Pleomorphic lobular carcinoma in situ: imaging features, upgrade rate, and clinical outcomes. AJR. 2018;211:462–7.

7. Rageth CJ, O'Flynn EAM, Pinker K, et al. Second international consensus conference on lesions of uncertain malignant potential in the breast (B3 lesions). Breast Cancer Res Treat. 2019;174:279–96.

8. Dawn Forester N, Lowes S, Mitchell E, Twiddy M. High risk (B3) breast lesions: what is the incidence of malignancy for individual lesion subtypes? A systematic review and meta-analysis. Eur J Surg Oncol. 2019;45:519–27.

9. Nakhlis F, Harrison BT, Giess CS, et al. Evaluating the rate of upgrade to invasive breast cancer and/or ductal carcinoma in situ following a core biopsy diagnosis of *non-classic* lobular carcinoma in situ. Ann Surg Oncol. 2019;26:55–61.

10. Shamir ER, Chen YY, Chu T, et al. Pleomorphic and florid lobular carcinoma in situ variants of the breast: a clinicopathologic study of 85 cases with and without invasive carcinoma from a single academic center. Am J Surg Pathol. 2019;43:399–408.

11. Shousha S, Eusebi V, Lester S. Paget disease of the nipple. In: Lakhani SR, Ellis IO, Schnitt SJ, et al., editors. WHO classification of tumours of the breast. Lyon: International Agency for Research on Cancer; 2012. p. 152–3.

12. Shousha S. Glandular Paget's disease of the nipple. Histopathology. 2007;50:812–4.

13. Soler T, Lerin A, Serrano T, et al. Pigmented Paget disease of the breast nipple with underlying infiltrating carcinoma: a case report and review of the literature. Am J Dermatopathol. 2011;33:e54–7.

14. Toker C. Clear cells of the nipple epidermis. Cancer. 1970;25:601–10.

15. Saeed D, Shousha S. Toker cells of the nipple are commonly associated with underlying sebaceous glands but not with lactiferous ducts. J Clin Pathol. 2014;67:1010–2.

16. Lee H-W, Kim TE, Cho SY, et al. Invasive Paget disease of the breast: 20 years of experience at a single institution. Hum Pathol. 2014;45:2480–7.

17. Collins LC, Schnitt SJ. Papillary lesions of the breast. Selected diagnostic and management issues. Histopathology. 2008;52:20–9.

18. Rakha E. Papillary carcinomas. In: Shousha S, editor. Breast pathology. Problematic issues. Switzerland: Springer International Publishing; 2017. p. 137–52.

19. Rakha EA, Varga Z, Elsheik S, Ellis IO. High-grade encapsulated papillary carcinoma of the breast: an under-recognised entity. Histopathology. 2015;66:740–6.

20. Silver SA, Tavassoli FA. Pleomorphic carcinoma of the breast: clinico-pathological analysis of 25 cases of an unusual high-grade phenotype of ductal carcinoma. Histopathology. 2000;36:505–14.

21. Nguyen CV, et al. Pleomorphic ductal carcinoma of the breast: predictors of decreased overall survival. Am J Surg Pathol. 2010;34:486–93.

22. Zhao J, et al. Clinicopathologic characteristics of pleomorphic carcinoma of the breast. Virchows Arch. 2010;456:31–7.

23. Shousha S. Pleomorphic invasive ductal carcinoma of the breast in a patient with Huntington's disease. Case Rep Pathol. 2014;214:979137. https://doi.org/10.1155/2014/979137.

24. Sastre-Garau X, Jouve M, Asselain B, et al. Infiltrating lobular carcinoma of the breast. Clinicopathologic analysis of 975 cases with reference to data on conservative therapy and metastatic pattern. Cancer. 1996;77:113–20.

25. Peiro G, Bornstein BA, Connolly JL, et al. The influence of infiltrating lobular carcinoma on the outcome of patients treated with breast-conserving surgery and radiation therapy. Breast Cancer Res Treat. 2000;59:49–54.

26. Evans WP, Warren Burchenne LJ, et al. Invasive lobular carcinoma of the breast: mammographic characteristics and computer-aided detection. Radiology. 2002;225:182–9.

27. Dejode M, Sagan C, Campion L, et al. Pure tubular carcinoma of the breast and sentinel lymph node biopsy: a retrospective multi-institutional study of 234 cases. Eur J Surg Oncol. 2013;39:248–54.

28. Poirier E, Drsbiens C, Poirier B, et al. Characteristics and long-term survival of patients diagnosed with pure tubular carcinoma of the breast. J Surg Oncol. 2018;117:1137–43.

29. Jorns JM, Thomas DG, Healy PN, et al. Estrogen receptor expression is high but is of lower intensity in tubular carcinoma than in well differentiated invasive ductal carcinoma. Arch Pathol Lab Med. 2014;138:1507–13.

30. Vo T, Xing Y, Meric-Bernstam F, et al. Long-term outcomes in patients with mucinous, medullary, tubular and invasive ductal carcinomas after lumpectomy. Am J Surg. 2007;194:527–31.

31. Page DL, Dixon JM, Anderson TJ, et al. Invasive cribriform carcinoma of the breast. Histopathology. 1983;7:525–36.

32. Venable JG, Schwartz AM, Silverberg SG. Infiltrating cribriform carcinoma of the breast: a distinctive clinicopathologic entity. Hum Pathol. 1990;21:333–8.

33. Shousha S, Schoenfeld S, Moss A, et al. Light and electron microscopic study of an invasive cribriform carcinoma with extensive microcalcification developing in a breast with silicone augmentation. Ultrastruct Pathol. 1994;18:519–23.

34. Dieci MV, Orvieto E, Dominici M, et al. Rare breast cancer subtypes: histological, molecular, and clinical peculiarities. Oncologist. 2014;19:805–13.

35. Damfeh AB, Carley AL, Striobel JM, et al. WT1 immunoreactivity in breast carcinoma: selective expression in pure and mixed mucinous subtypes. Mod Pathol. 2008;21:1217–23.

36. Dadmanesh F, Peterse JL, Sapino A, et al. Lymphoepithelioma-like carcinoma of the breast: lack of evidence of Epstein-Barr virus infection. Histopathology. 2001;38:54–61.

37. Shousha S, Anscombe O, McFarlane T. All benign and malignant apocrine breast lesions over-express claudin 1 and 3 and are negative for claudin 4. Pathol Oncol Res. 2019. https://doi.org/10.1007/s12253-019-00662-9.

38. Vranic S, Tawfik O, Palazzo J, et al. EGFR and HER-2/neu expression in invasive apocrine carcinoma of the breast. Mod Pathol. 2010;23:644–53.

39. Dellapasqua S, Maisonneuve P, Viale G, et al. Immunohistochemically defined subtypes and outcome of apocrine breast cancer. Clin Breast Cancer. 2013;13:95–102.

40. Tse G, Moriya T, Niu Y. Invasive papillary carcinoma. In: Lakhani SR, Ellis IO, Schnitt SJ, et al., editors. WHO classification of tumours of the breast. Lyon: International Agency for Research on Cancer; 2012. p. 64.

41. Guo X, Chen L, Lang R, et al. Invasive micropapillary carcinoma of the breast. Association of pathologic features with lymph node metastasis. Am J Clin Pathol. 2006;126:140–6.

42. Yang Y-T, Liu B-B, Zhang X, Fu L. Invasive micropapillary carcinoma of the breast. An update. Arch Pathol Lab Med. 2016;140:799–805.

43. Pettinato G, Manivel CJ, Panico L, et al. Invasive micropapillary carcinoma of the breast. Clinicopathologic study of 62 cases of a poorly recognized variant with highly aggressive behaviour. Am J Clin Pathol. 2004;121:857–66.

44. Tan PH, Schnitt SJ, van de Vijver MJ, et al. Papillary and neuroendocrine breast lesions: the WHO stance. Histopathology. 2015;66:761–70.

45. Rosen LE, Gattuso P. Neuroendocrine tumors of the breast. Arch Pathol Lab Med. 2017;141:1577–81.

46. Hayes MM, Seidman JD, Ashto MA. Glycogen-rich clear cell carcinoma of the breast. A clinicopathologic study of 21 cases. Am J Surg Pathol. 1995;19(8):904–11.

47. Zhou Z, Kinslow CJ, Hibshoosh H, et al. Clinical features, survival and prognostic factors of glycogen-rich clear cell carcinoma (GRCC) of the breast in the U.S. population. J Clin Med. 2019;8(2). pii: E246. https://doi.org/10.3390/jcm8020246.

48. Guan B, Wang H, Cao S, et al. Lipid-rich carcinoma of the breast. Clinicopathologic analysis of 17 cases. Ann Diagn Pathol. 2011;15:225–32.

49. Rakha EA, Coimbra NDM, Hodi Z, et al. Immunoprofile of metaplastic carcinomas of the breast. Histopathology. 2017;70:975–85.

50. Rosen PP, Ernsberger D. Low grade adenosquamous carcinoma. A variant of metaplastic mammary carcinoma. Am J Surg Pathol. 1987;11:351–8.

51. Wargotz ES, Norris HJ. Metaplastic carcinoma of the breast. I. Matrix-producing carcinoma. Hum Pathol. 1989;20:628–35.
52. Kusafuka K, Muramatsu K, Kasami M, et al. Cartilaginous features in matrix-producing carcinoma of the breast: four cases report with histo-chemical and immunohistochemical analysis of matrix molecules. Mod Pathol. 2008;21:1282–92.
53. Downs-Kelly E, Nayeemuddin KM, Albarracin C, et al. Matrix-producing carcinoma of the breast. An aggressive subtype of metaplastic carcinoma. Am J Surg Pathol. 2009;33:534–41.
54. Ro JY, Silva EG, Gallager HS, et al. Adenoid cystic carcinoma of the breast. Hum Pathol. 1987;18:1276–81.
55. Poling JS, Yonescu R, Subhawong AP, et al. MYB labelling by immuno-histochemistry is more sensitive for breast adenoid cystic carcinoma than MYB labelling by FISH. Am J Surg Pathol. 2017;41:973–9.
56. Del Castillo M, Chibon F, Arnould L, et al. Secretory breast carcinoma. A histopathologic and genomic spectrum characterized by a joint specific *ETV6-NTRK3* fusion. Am J Surg Pathol. 2015;39:1458–67.
57. Rancoroli F, Lamovec J, Zidar A, Eusebi V. Acinic cell-like carcinoma of the breast. Virchows Arch. 1996;429:69–74.
58. Foschini MP, Morandi L, Asioli S, et al. The morphological spectrum of salivary gland type tumours of the breast. Pathology. 2017;49:215–27.
59. Geyer FC, Berman SH, Marchio C, et al. Genetic analysis of microglan-dular adenosis and acinic cell carcinomas of the breast provides evidence for the existence of a low-grade triple-negative breast neoplasia family. Mod Pathol. 2017;30:69–84.
60. Awamleh AA, Gudi M, Shousha S. Malignant adenomyoepithelioma of the breast with lymph node metastasis: a detailed immunohistochemical study. Case Rep Pathol. 2012;2012:305858.
61. Ahmadi N, Negahban S, Aledavood A, et al. Malignant adenomyoepithe-lioma of the breast: a review. Breast J. 2015;21:291–6.
62. Baum JE, Sung K-J, Tran H, et al. Mammary epithelial-myoepithelial carcinoma. Report of case with KRAS and AK3CA mutations by next-generation sequencing. Int J Surg Pathol. 2019;27:441–5.
63. Buza N, Zekry N, Charpin C, et al. Myoepithelial carcinoma of the breast: a clinicopathological and immunohistochemical study of 15 diagnosti-cally challenging cases. Virchows Arch. 2010;457:337–45.
64. Salarieh A, Sneige N. Breast carcinoma arising in microglandular adeno-sis. A review of the literature. Arch Pathol Lab Med. 2007;131:1397–9.
65. Elston CW, Ellis IO. Pathological prognostic factors in breast cancer. I. The value of histological grade in breast cancer: experience from a large study with long term follow up. Histopathology. 1991;19:403–10.
66. Jimenez RE, Bongers S, Bouwman D, Segel M, Visscher DW. Clinico-pathologic significance of ductal carcinoma in situ in breast core needle biopsies with invasive cancer. Am J Surg Pathol. 2000;24:123–8.

67. Pu RT, Schott AF, Sturtz DE, et al. Pathologic features of breast cancer associated with complete response to neoadjuvant chemotherapy. Importance of tumor necrosis. Am J Surg Pathol. 2005;29:354–8.

68. Loi S, Michiels S, Salgado R, et al. Tumor infiltrating lymphocytes are prognostic in triple negative breast cancer and predictive for trastuzumab benefit in early breast cancer: results from the FinHER trial. Ann Oncol. 2014;25:1544–50.

69. Pruneri G, Vingiani A, Bagnardi V, et al. Clinical validity of tumor-infiltrating lymphocytes analysis in patients with triple-negative breast cancer. Ann Oncol. 2016;27:249–56.

70. Savas P, Salgado R, Denkert C, et al. Clinical relevance of host immunity in breast cancer: from TILs to the clinic. Nat Rev Clin Oncol. 2016;13:228–41.

71. Denkert C, von Minckwitz G, Darb-Esfahani S, et al. Tumour-infiltrating lymphocytes and prognosis in different subtypes of breast cancer: a pooled analysis of 3771 patients treated with neoadjuvant therapy. Lancet Oncol. 2018;19:40–50.

72. Salgado R, Denkert C, Demaria S, et al. The evaluation of tumor-infiltrating lymphocytes (TILs) in breast cancer: recommendations by an International TILs working group 2014. Ann Oncol. 2015;26: 259–71.

73. Lester SC, Bose S, Chen Y-Y, Connolly JL, de Baca ME, Fitzgibbons PL, et al. Protocol for the examination of specimens from patients with invasive carcinoma of the breast. Arch Pathol Lab Med. 2009;133: 1515–38.

74. Shousha S. Oestrogen receptor status of breast carcinoma. Allred/H score conversion. Histopathology. 2004;53:346–7.

75. Wolff AC, Hammond MEH, Allison KH, et al. Human epidermal growth factor receptor 2 testing in breast cancer. American Society of Clinical Oncology/College of American Pathologists clinical practice guideline focused update. J Clin Oncol. 2018;36:2105–22.

76. Koh YW, Lee HJ, Lee JW, et al. Dual-color silver-enhanced *in situ* hybridization for assessing *HER2* gene amplification in breast cancer. Mod Pathol. 2011;24:794–800.

77. Marchio C, Dell'Orto P, Annaratone L, et al. The dilemma of HER2 double-equivocal breast carcinoma. Genomic profiling and implications for treatment. Am J Surg Pathol. 2018;42:1190–200.

78. Liberman L, Zakowski M, Avery S, Hudis C, Morris EA, Abramson AF, LaTrenta LR, Glassman JR, Dershaw DD. Complete percutaneous excision of infiltrating carcinoma at stereotactic breast biopsy: how can tumor size be assessed? AJR. 1999;173:1315–22.

79. Liberman L. Percutaneous imaging-guided core breast biopsy: state of the art at the millennium. AJR. 2000;174:1191–9.

80. Shousha S, Sinnett HD. Chest wall tumors presenting as breast lumps. Breast J. 2004;10:150–3.

81. Jozefczyk MA, Rosen PP. Vascular tumors of the breast. II. Perilobular hemangiomas and hemangiomas. Am J Surg Pathol. 1985;9:491–503.
82. Biswas T, Tang P, Muhs A, Ling M. Angiosarcoma of the breast. A rare clinicopathological entity. Am J Clin Oncol. 2009;32:582–6.
83. Strobbe LJA, Peterse HL, van Tinteren H, Wijnmaalen A, Rutgers EJT. Angiosarcoma of the breast after conservation therapy for invasive cancer, the incidence and outcome. An unforseen sequela. Breast Cancer Res Treat. 1998;47:101–9.
84. Wijnmaalen A, van Ooijen B, van Geel BN, Henzen-Logmans SC, Treurniet-Donker AD. Angiosarcoma of the breast following lumpectomy, axillary lymph node dissection, and radiotherapy for primary breast cancer: three case reports and a review of the literature. Int J Radiat Oncol Biol Phys. 1993;26:135–9.
85. Rosen PP, Kimmel M, Ernsberger D. Mammary angiosarcoma. The prognostic significance of tumor differentiation. Cancer. 1988;62:2145–51.
86. Fineberg S, Rosen PP. Cutaneous angiosarcoma and atypical vascular lesions of the skin and breast after radiation therapy for breast carcinoma. Am J Clin Pathol. 1994;102:757–63.
87. Parham DM, Fisher C. Angiosarcoma of the breast developing post radiotherapy. Histopathology. 1997;31:189–95.
88. Mentzei T, Schildhaus HU, Palmedo G, et al. Postradiation cutaneous angiosarcoma after treatment of breast carcinoma is characterized by MYC amplification in contrast to atypical vascular lesions after radiotherapy and control cases: clinicopathological, immunohistochemical and molecular analysis of 66 cases. Mod Pathol. 2012;25:75–85.
89. Nascimento AF, Raut CP, Fletcher CDM. Primary angiosarcoma of the breast. Clinicopathologic analysis of 49 cases, suggesting that grade is not prognostic. Am J Surg Pathol. 2008;32:1896–904.
90. Wang XY, Jakowski J, Tawfik OW, Thomas PA, Fan F. Angiosarcoma of the breast: a clinicopathologic analysis of cases from the last 10 years. Ann Diagn Pathol. 2009;13:147–50.
91. Kotton DN, Muse VV, Nishino M. Case 202012: a 63-year-old woman with dyspnea and rapidly progressive respiratory failure. N Engl J Med. 2012;366:259–69.
92. Leibl S, Moinfar F. Mammary NOS-Type sarcoma with CD10 expression. A rare entity with features of myoepithelial differentiation. Am J Surg Pathol. 2006;30:450–6.
93. Callery CD, Rosen PP, Kinne DW. Sarcoma of the breast. A study of 32 patients with reappraisal of classification and therapy. Ann Surg. 1985;201:527–32.
94. Gutman H, Pollock RE, Ross MI, Benjamin RS, Johnston DA, Janjan NA, Ramsdahl MM. Sarcoma of the breast: implications for extent of therapy. The M.D. Anderson experience. Surgery. 1994;116:505–9.
95. Silver SA, Tavassoli FA. Primary osteogenic sarcoma of the breast. A clinicopathologic analysis of 50 cases. Am J Surg Pathol. 1998;22:925–33.

96. Pendlebury SC, Bilous M, Langlands AO. Sarcomas following radiation therapy: a report of three cases and a review of the literature. Int J Radiat Oncol Biol Phys. 1995;31:405–10.

97. Brogi E, Harris NL. Lymphomas of the breast: pathology and clinical behavior. Semin Oncol. 1999;26:357–64.

98. Lin Y, Govindan R, Hess JL. Malignant hematopoietic breast tumors. Am J Clin Pathol. 1997;107:177–86.

99. Topalovski M, Crisan D, Mattson JC. Lymphoma of the breast. A clinicopathologic study of primary and secondary cases. Arch Pathol Lab Med. 1999;123:1208–18.

100. Mattia AR, Ferry JA, Harris NL. Breast lymphoma. A B-cell spectrum including the low grade B-cell lymphoma of mucosa associated lymphoid tissue. Am J Surg Pathol. 1993;17:574–87.

101. Arber DA, Simpson JF, Weiss LM, Rappaport H. Non-Hodgkin's lymphoma involving the breast. Am J Surg Pathol. 1994;18:288–95.

102. Borbow LG, Richards MA, Happerfield LC, Diss TC, Isaacson PG, Lammie GA, Millis RR. Breast lymphoma: a clinicopathologic review. Hum Pathol. 1993;24:274–8.

103. Martinelli G, Ryan G, Seymour JF, Nassi L, Steffanoni S, Alietti A, Calabrese L, Pruneri G, Santoro L, Kuper-Hommel M, Tsang R, Zinzani PL, Taghian A, Zucca E, Cavalli F. Primary follicular and marginal-zone lymphoma of the breast: clinical features, prognostic factors and outcome: a study by the international extranodal lymphoma study group. Ann Oncol. 2009;20:1993–9.

104. Miranda RN, Talwalker SS, Manning JT, Meddeiros LJ. Anaplastic large cell lymphoma involving the breast. A clinicopathologic study of 6 cases and review of the literature. Arch Pathol Lab Med. 2009;133:1383–90.

105. Aguilera NSI, Tavassoli FA, Chu W-S, Abbondanzo SL. T-cell lymphoma presenting in the breast: a histologic, immunophenotypic and molecular genetic study of four cases. Mod Pathol. 2000;13: 599–605.

106. Gualco G, Chioato L, Harrington WJ, Weiss L, Bacchi CE. Primary and secondary T-cell lymphomas of the breast. Clinicopathologic features of 11 cases. Appl Immunohistochem Mol Morphol. 2009;17:301–6.

107. Meis JM, Butler JJ, Osborne BM. Hodgkin's disease involving the breast and chest wall. Cancer. 1986;57:1859–65.

108. D'Amore ESG, Wick MR, Geisinger KR, Frizzera G. Primary malignant lymphoma arising in postmastectomy lymphedema. Another facet of Stewart-Treves syndrome. Am J Surg Pathol. 1990;14:456–63.

109. Ryan G, Martinelli G, Kuper-Hommel M, et al. Primary diffuse large B-cell lymphoma of the breast: prognostic factors and outcomes of a study by the International Extranodal Lymphoma Study Group. Ann Oncol. 2008;19:233–41.

110. Giardini R, Piccolo C, Rilke F. Primary non-Hodgkin's lymphoma of the female breast. Cancer. 1992;69:725–35.
111. Ebner PJ, Liu A, Gould DJ, Patel KM. Breast implant associated anaplastic large cell lymphoma, a systematic review and in-depth evaluation of the current understanding. J Surg Oncol. 2019;120:573–7.
112. DeLair DF, Corben AD, Catalano JP, et al. Non-mammary metastases to the breast and axilla: a study of 85 cases. Mod Pathol. 2013;26: 343–9.

Dealing with the Excised Specimen

6

Introduction

Once a core biopsy is given a B3, 4 or 5, indicating the presence of a slightly [3] or markedly [4] worrying lesion or a frankly malignant one [5], an action has to be taken. This used to be surgical excision in almost all cases of B3 and 5, as B4 usually need a repeat core biopsy. Currently, many B3 lesions are managed by a vacuum assisted excision, which does not need hospital admission even as a day surgery case. The rest of the B3 lesions and almost all B5 lesions will need surgery. This would vary from a wide local excision, in which the lesion may or may not need to be localised before surgery, to mastectomy. In malignant cases, both procedures might be preceded by 'neo-adjuvant' chemo or hormone therapy. A surgical lymph node procedure is also usually needed in malignant cases which may be in the form of sentinel node biopsy, node sampling or axillary clearance.

Vacuum Assisted Excision

A recent consensus conference has recommended using vacuum assisted excision (VAE), rather than open surgical excision, for managing a variety of B3 lesions diagnosed by core or vacuum assisted biopsy [1]. These lesions include flat epithelial atypia; classical in situ lobular neoplasia if the lesion was visible on imaging and is not of the pleomorphic or florid type; small benign

© Springer Nature Switzerland AG 2020
S. Shousha, *Breast Pathology in Clinical Practice*, In Clinical
Practice, https://doi.org/10.1007/978-3-030-42386-5_6

intraduct papillomas with no atypia, radial scars/complex sclerosing lesions with no atypia [1] and mucocele-like lesions [2]. The aim is to completely remove these lesions and to exclude the presence of more advanced lesions. The procedure is not recommended for B3 lesions showing atypical ductal hyperplasia, spindle cell lesions or those suggestive of phyllodes tumour. On the other hand, the procedure is sometimes used, using wider needles, to remove B2 lesions (like small fibroadenomas), or even small malignant lesions

Like core and vacuum assisted biopsies, the material removed is placed immediately in formalin by the Radiologist after removal. Two separate specimens are usually received: a first and a second round specimens. The former is taken from the site of the previous biopsy which may have been indicated by a marker clip left behind in the breast after doing a first line vacuum assisted biopsy. This round will include what remains of the target lesion. The second, outer, round of specimens is taken from the surrounding tissue to help establishing the complete removal of the lesion, which is usually what is hoped if the lesion is around 15 mm or less.

The amount of tissue received will depend on the size of the target lesion and the gauge of the needle used which can vary from a relatively thin 14 to a much wider bore needle of 8 or 7 gauge. The 11 gauge needles are the most commonly used in our institution. All tissue is processed usually in more than one cassette depending on the number and size of tissue fragments removed. Three levels are routinely cut from each paraffin block and stained with H&E, but more levels may be needed, particularly if the biopsy was done for microcalcification and these were not found in the original three levels.

The outcome of the procedure is reported in a way similar to surgical excision which does not need a 'B' code. The report should clearly state whether the lesion is benign or malignant, and if benign whether atypia is present or not. Lesions with atypia will need follow up. Malignant lesions will require surgery. Sometimes no residual tumour is found in the follow up surgical excision and determining the size of the lesion, whether in situ or invasive, would have to be decided by measuring the lesion in the vacuum biopsy.

Other Excision Biopsies

Good fixation is essential for proper diagnosis. In our department we prefer to receive all excised breast specimens fresh in plastic bags, immediately after surgical excision whenever this is feasible and in the absence of any suspected infections. The specimen is registered, given a laboratory number, and the Pathologist in charge is called to deal with it. For biopsies coming from other hospitals we ask the surgeons to immerse it in an adequate amount of formalin and send it to us as soon as possible where it is dealt with immediately. If there is going to be a delay, for example cases done late before a week end or a Holiday, we advice slicing mastectomy specimens to expose the tumour, before immersing in formalin. The specimen container should be big enough to accommodate the specimen without distorting it, and must be clearly labeled with the patient identity and side and type of specimen. It should be accompanied by a request form detailing the patient's name, date of birth, hospital number, clinicians name, location, date of request and relevant clinical history. The information written on the specimen container is checked with that on the request form, particularly as regards the patient's name and type and side of the biopsy. Any tissue left after sampling a specimen is retained for 4–5 weeks post authorization of the report.

Wire Guided Biopsies

Inserting a 'hooked wire' in impalpable screen detected lesions under x-ray or ultrasound examination by radiologists is the most commonly used method for localising these lesions prior to surgical removal. The surgeons usually x-ray the excised specimen before sending it to the Histology lab to ensure that the radiologically abnormal area has been removed (Fig. 6.1). In this way, the surgeon can undertake further excisions if the x-ray does not confirm the presence of the lesion in the biopsy or when the abnormality reaches the excision margin. The x-ray is usually carried out in theatre using a faxitron.

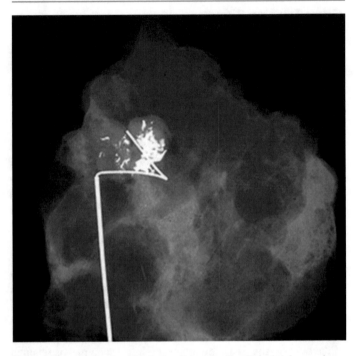

Fig. 6.1 Specimen x-ray with the localizing needle within the abnormal area where the calcification is present

The biopsies are received with the wires still attached and with attached sutures indicating the orientation of the specimen; usually a long suture indicating lateral, short superior and loop anterior. This would help identifying the anterior and posterior surfaces of the specimen, as well as the lateral, medial, superior and inferior surfaces. We discourage embedding metal clips for orientation, as these can be difficult to remove and may lead to underlying tissue damage. Instead metal clips can be successfully attached to the sutures for visual assessment of the specimen by x-ray in the theatre. Sometimes the sutures attached do not make sense, for example the superior suture is attached opposite the lateral one. In this situation, the surgeon should be contacted and asked to provide the correct orientation.

The biopsy is described, weighed, measured in three dimensions and the wire, or sometimes multiple wires, are gently removed. The specimen is then inked with different coloured inks to indicate the different surfaces. Abundant amount of ink should be applied using a brush or cotton wool mounted on sticks. Four colours are used to indicate anterior and posterior, or superior and inferior surfaces as well as lateral and medial (Fig. 6.2). In larger specimens, more colours can be used to indicate other surfaces. A few drops of 1% acetic acid or absolute alcohol are added to the inked areas to help the adherence of the ink to the specimen surfaces. Allow a couple of minutes for the ink to dry and remove excess ink with blotting paper.

There are two different ways of cutting up the specimen. Some centres prefer to cut the specimen horizontally. This has the advantage of providing a 'panoramic' view of the whole specimen in a way similar to that seen in an x-ray, hence allowing identification of the lesion in its entirety and its relationship to the radial margins. This method also helps identifying multiple lesions and

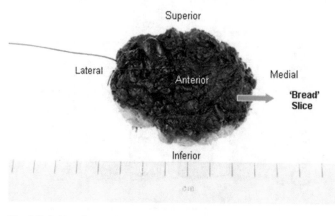

Fig. 6.2 Inking the specimen with a different colour for each margin, before slicing it

their relationship to each other. However, cutting horizontally can be difficult to control and the relationship of the tumour to the anterior and posterior margins may not be possible assess.

The other method of cutting up specimens is the 'bread slicing' method where the specimen is cut vertically into approximately 4 mm-thick slices along its long axis, starting from the narrowest end of the specimen. This is the method we use in our Lab as well as in most other Labs. In this way all margins can be examined microscopically. The actual size of the lesion can be estimated by multiplying the number of slices involved with the thickness of each slice, provided that the calculated size is more than the tumour size in a given section.

For small specimens, weighing 25 g or less, all slices are processed. For larger specimens, the first and last slice are processed as well as all slices containing obvious tumour tissue and the immediately adjacent slices, including the margins nearest to the tumour (Fig. 6.3). Samples are also taken from other slices with obvious gross abnormality. If the biopsy contains no palpable abnormality, all slices with grossly abnormal looking areas are processed, as well as randomly sampled ones. If the biopsy contains more than one obvious tumour, each is recorded, measured and clearly labeled separately.

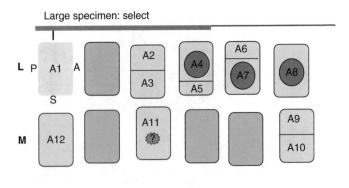

Fig. 6.3 Tissue selection for processing from a large specimen. The red colour indicates the tumour, while the green coloured area in A11 indicates another grossly abnormal area. The yellow coloured slices are the ones that are going to be processed

If the excision was undertaken for microcalcification or for an impalpable lesion, rather than a well-defined tumour, it is advisable to x-ray the slices, if that is possible and if not all the specimen is going to be processed. X-raying can be carried out in a departmental Faxtron, if available, or in the Radiology department. This helps to identify the slice(s) containing the calcification that or radiological abnormality correspond to that seen in the mammogram (Fig. 6.4). All slices containing radiological abnormalities and their adjacent ones are processed together with any other slices that may appear macroscopically suspicious. This would include the site of any previous recent needle aspiration or core/vacuum biopsies which is usually indicated by an area of

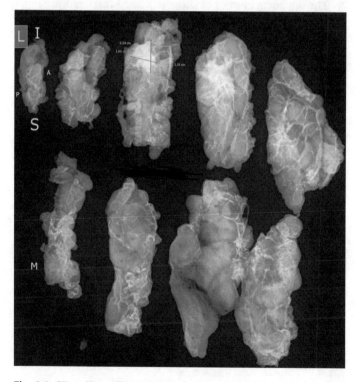

Fig. 6.4 Slices X-ray. The tumour is in slices 3 and 4, but there are other abnormal-looking areas that have to be processed. Also note how the specimen outline is quite irregular

haemorrhage or by the presence of a marker that was introduced at the time of the original core/vacuum biopsy.

Many cases of invasive lobular carcinoma will present in the form of a diffuse thickening, rather than a well-defined mass, and satellite lesions adjacent to the main tumour may be present, some being impalpable. Thorough sampling is especially required in these cases, particularly from the excision margins, to assess complete removal.

If pure DCIS is suspected, usually with a greyish coarse granular appearance, sometimes with 'comedo' necrotic streaks, all obvious abnormal tissue has to be processed to avoid missing a small focus of invasive carcinoma.

The minimum number of slices processed from each specimen is six, but the total number will depend on the size of the biopsy and the extent of abnormalities seen. Each slice is processed in a separate cassette marked with the case number and an additional serial number which we also recorded in a special map (Fig. 6.5) or on the corresponding slice x-ray if that was done. We also use a separate form listing the cassette number, the source of the sample taken and the number of tissue pieces in each cassette (Fig. 6.6). If a slice suspected of containing lesion is too large for the cassette, a mega cassette is used (Fig. 6.7), or the slice is divided and processed in two normal sized cassettes. The mega cassette has the advantage of providing an overall view of the tumour and surrounding margins (Fig. 6.8). The site of all blocks in the specimen must be carefully noted in the block details dictated during dissection and recorded in the map and the cassettes list. Fat is not trimmed off the slices, as ink usually seeps through the fat down to the surface of the more firm tissue underneath, which would give a false impression of the actual surgical resection margin if the fat is removed.

If a second specimen is received from the same breast, either because the specimen radiograph of the first biopsy did not confirm the complete removal of the mammographic abnormality, or because the surgeon was able to feel a suspicious area in the cavity after removing the first biopsy, the second specimen is treated in the same way as described above.

It must be added here that not all biopsies have an ideal shape with regular margins. Biopsies with irregular or friable margins are commonly received (Figs. 6.4 and 6.9). All efforts should be

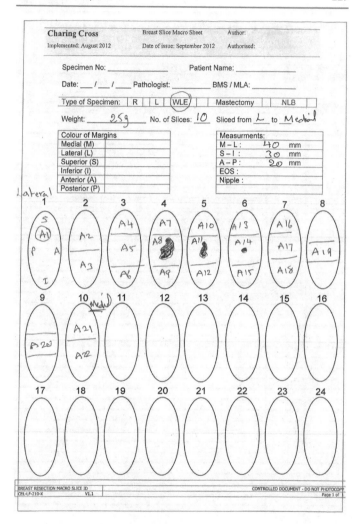

Fig. 6.5 An example of a completed map

made to delineate each margin and to mention in the gross description any difficulty encountered doing this or the fact that the specimen was friable and received with separate pieces of fat in the pot (which should be processed separately), so that this can be taken into consideration when the microscopic report is made.

**GENERAL MACROSCOPIC DESCRIPTION TEMPLATE FOR
MULTIBOCK CASSETTES, TO BE ATTACHED TO REQUEST FORM**

SPECIMEN NO		DATE	
PATIENT NAME		PATHOLOGIST	

BLOCK	PIECES	DESCRIPTION and CUTTING REQUEST

Fig. 6.6 The form used for listing the samples taken from the specimen, the number of the cassette containing the sample, the site from which the sample is taken and the number of pieces of tissue in each cassette

The cassettes containing the slices are kept in 10% neutral buffered formalin overnight and then processed the following day, with the stained slides usually available for examination within 48 h.

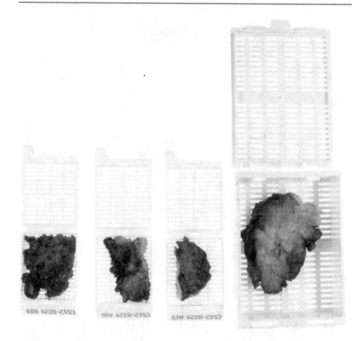

Fig. 6.7 A picture of the small and large (Mega) cassettes

As a routine, frozen section examinations are not performed on these lesions or on biopsy margins. The lesions, if they are identifiable by the naked eye, can be small and sometimes multifocal. A complete accurate diagnosis necessitates microscopic examination of properly processed sections of all abnormal areas of the biopsy and their adjacent margins.

Wide Local Excision Biopsies and Therapeutic Mammoplasties

Wide local excision biopsies are the most commonly performed operations for palpable lesions, whether screen-detected or symptomatic. In therapeutic mammoplasties, which are much less commonly done, the whole breast quadrant containing the

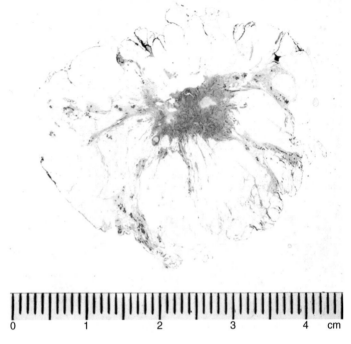

Fig. 6.8 Mega section. The tumour and surrounding margins are clearly visualized

Fig. 6.9 Wire guided biopsy with irregular margins

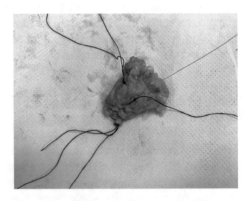

tumour is excised. An essential requirement for the success of either operation is to ensure the complete removal of all malignant tissue. Theses specimens are dealt with basically in a similar way to that described under wire guided biopsy. The margins are inked and the specimen is sliced in the same manner. The lesions in these specimens are relatively large and can be identified by the naked eye. It is usually useful to review the mammogram of the case to identify the site of the lesion and whether there is one or more than one lesion in the specimen. The margins are thoroughly sampled and all slices with obvious tumour or other abnormality are processed together with the adjacent ones (Fig. 6.3). At some centres, frozen sections of the biopsy margins or cytology imprints of its surface are done for that purpose. We do not advocate using these time- consuming intra-operative procedures as they use less than optimal microscopic methods for diagnosis and are done under pressure while the patient is still anesthetised and the surgeon waiting for the result to proceed with the operation.

Cavity Wall, Margins, Shaves and Tumour Bed Biopsies

Most surgeons remove extra strips of breast tissue from the wall of the cavity left in the breast after doing a wide local excision, whether wire guided or not, to ensure complete removal of the lesion. They give them different names, as seen in the heading above, but they are all dealt with in the same way. Usually there is more than one biopsy, each received separately with an indication of the side from which it was taken, e.g., medial, lateral, etc. The surgeon usually marks the inner or outer surface of the specimens with a stitch. The specimens are weighed measured and the surfaces inked. I personally ink just one surface indicating the new, outer, margin of the specimen, as identified by the stitch. The other, inner surface, can also be inked with a different colour. The specimen is sliced perpendicularly across its long axis into short strips, around 4 mm thick, so that the inner and outer, painted, surfaces are included in each section. All slices are processed.

Each biopsy is reported separately. If tumour tissue is identified in a biopsy, the type of tumour, whether in situ or invasive, is reported as well as its size and distance from the outer margin.

Re-excision Biopsies

A re-excision biopsy may have to be carried out after a wire local-isation or a wide local excision biopsy, if microscopic examination shows tumour tissue at the excision margin. These are usually small specimens as those described in the previous section and are dealt with in the same way. If the re-excision specimen is too large to be totally processed, samples have to be taken from selected areas particularly from around the previous biopsy site and from any other grossly abnormal area, as well as from the new excision margins to ensure complete removal of any residual tumour tissue. The likelihood of finding small foci of residual tumour increases with the increase in the number of cavity wall slices examined [3].

Most of these biopsies are carried out because of the presence of foci of DCIS at the margins. It is not unusual for a palpable invasive tumour to be surrounded, for a variable distance, by impalpable DCIS foci that can be left behind. Also, in wire local-isation biopsies, tumour tissue may extend beyond the mammo-graphic abnormality and the margins of the biopsy. The more DCIS elements present in and adjacent to the invasive tumour, the more likely that similar foci will be present beyond the excision margins; and these are the cases that have been shown to be more prone to recurrence, possibly because of incomplete removal in the first instance [4].

In some cases, a third operation, usually a mastectomy, is inev-itable because of the presence of widespread DCIS.

Lumpectomy Specimens

These are usually done for benign lesions, most commonly fibro-adenomas, which are removed with variable amount of 'normal' breast tissue around them. The biopsy is described, weighed, measured and its surface inked, as sometimes the lesion might turn out to be a phyllodes tumour or an unexpected different benign or malignant lesion on microscopic examination. If orientation sutures are present, different colour inks are used as described above under wire localization biopsies.

According to its size, the specimen is either processed in its entirety, after being bisected, e.g. a small fibroadenoma, or selectively sampled after being sliced. The cut surface of the specimen should be described. Sampling must be directed mainly at the non-fatty areas of the biopsy, as the likelihood of finding any epithelial lesions within pure adipose tissue is extremely low [5].

Mastectomy Specimens

The specimen is weighed, measured and described macroscopically as a right/left breast with/without an axillary tail. Note whether any attached chest wall tissue is present. The attached skin is measured (length and width) and examined for signs of previous operations or any other abnormality. If a prior biopsy site is present, the scar is described (recent, healed), measured and its location in the skin reported quadrant location in the breast. If present, the nipple is described particularly as regards the presence or absence of retraction or evidence of inflammation or ulceration.

The specimen is inked before slicing. All surfaces, posterior, anterior, superior and inferior, can be inked with four different colours. Alternatively, the posterior surface is inked with one colour and then the surface opposite the tumour, if it is palpable or its position is known, with a second different colour. A few drops of 1% acetic acid or absolute alcohol are added to the inked surfaces and allowed to dry in a couple of minutes, before removing the excess ink with blotting paper.

The specimen is then sliced. In some centres this is done horizontally for the reasons given above where local excisions are discussed. In our hospital, and most other institutions, the specimen is 'bread' sliced perpendicularly from one side to the other, with each slice being approximately 1 cm thick. I prefer to do the slicing from anterior to posterior to keep track of where exactly the lesion is in relation to the anterior surface and the nipple if present. Many Pathologists prefer to do the slicing from the deep aspect of the specimen outwards. The lesion(s) are identified and described particularly as regards their size, location and distance from the nearest margin. Tumours or the walls of previously excised biopsies are processed in their entirety if this is feasible. This is particularly important in DCIS cases, to ensure that a small invasive focus is not missed. Sections are also taken from any other abnormal areas as well as from the nipple. We do not take samples from the four breast quadrants if they appear normal. If lymph nodes are included in the specimen, these are dealt with as described below.

There is usually no problem in identifying large tumours because of their abnormal, usually greyish, colour and, usually hard, consistency. Smaller tumours may be difficult to identify. The surgeon should have mentioned in the request form the exact site of the tumour or tumours, if these were multiple. Some surgeons attach a suture to the skin covering the tumour(s) to help its identification by the Pathologist. If this information is not available, reviewing the mammogram in the Lab during, or before, dissection would help localising the lesion(s). The suspected slice can then be x-rayed, if x-raying facilities are available, to confirm the presence of the mammographic abnormality.

If there is no facilities to review the x-rays, thorough sampling of all abnormal, relatively harder, areas has to be carried out. In high grade DCIS, the presence of tiny foci oozing comedo necrotic material in a background of a greyish hard area, helps in pointing out the site of the lesion. It has been suggested that x-raying the slices of mastectomies carried out for extensive high grade DCIS, is advisable in order to locate the associated calcification and thus help sampling the specimen.

If lymph nodes are included in the specimen, these are dealt with as described in the section below.

'Prophylactic (risk-reducing) mastectomies' are dealt with in the same way, with samples taken from any suspicious areas, or in the absence of such areas, from various parts of the breast containing fibrous tissue

Axillary Lymph Node Specimens

Core Biopsy

Clinically palpable or radiologically abnormal lymph nodes are usually subjected to core biopsy or fine needle aspiration by the Radiologist at the time of taking the breast core biopsy. Lymph node core biopsies are dealt with in the same way as breast cores. Thus, three levels are cut and stained with H&E. These are usually sufficient to confirm the presence or absence of lymph node tissue in the specimen and whether there is or there is no evidence of metastasis. Immunohistochemistry for pancytokeratin is advisable if there are suspicious atypical cells particularly in cases of invasive lobular carcinoma.

Sentinel Node Biopsies

Sentinel lymph node biopsy is now considered the standard of care for axillary staging in patients with clinically and radiologically node negative invasive breast carcinoma [6]. The sentinel lymph node is the first node to which lymph drainage and metastasis from breast cancer occurs. It is usually situated in level I, but it could be in level II or III, intramammary, interpectoral, an internal mammary node or even a supraclavicular node [7]. The node is identified by injecting a radio-labeled isotope (usually technetium Tc 99m-labelled colloid) or a blue dye or both in the breast skin, and then locating the node surgically in the axilla either by a handheld probe that detects gamma rays emission and/or the blue dye colour.

Eighty five percent of patients have a single sentinel node with 15% having two or more [8]. It has been shown that in the hands of experienced surgeons, the sentinel node, because of its location at the forefront of all other draining nodes, reflects the true axillary lymph node status in 95% of appropriately selected patients (usually those with tumours less than 3 cm in diameter and clinically negative axilla) [8]. Thus, if the sentinel node is free of tumour, the patient can be spared further axillary dissection with its associated high morbidity. The procedure can be applied to patients who had neoadjuvant chemotherapy prior to or after their surgery [9].

Handling sentinel nodes detected by radioactive isotopes can be worrying for Laboratory staff and Pathologists. However, a Consensus Conference held in 2001 has analysed the available data and expressed no objections to the immediate processing of sentinel nodes as 'they contain radioactivity (that) results in a level of personal exposure that is a small fraction of the maximum allowable yearly dose' [7]. Also, The American Association of Directors of Anatomic and Surgical Pathology has advised that 'delaying the dealing with sentinel lymph nodes does not appear to be justified, but delaying processing primary tumour excision specimens may be considered because of the higher radioactivity levels in these specimens compared with the sentinel lymph node' [10]. However, monitoring the level of radiation in the laboratory and in the examined specimens is recommended as increased radioactivity in the submitted specimens has been noted in some institution over time [11]. If sentinel lymph nodes are dealt with while fresh, for example for frozen section examination, this should be done in a special area of the cut up room. Any contaminated material used (plastic bag containers and blades) should be disposed of in a special container according to specific guidelines drawn in accordance with the hospital's radiation safety policy. These safety issues do not arise if only blue dye is used for localisation, but the false negative rate would be higher (12% for a single agent and 6% for dual agents) [12].

The main goal of sentinel node examination is to detect macro-metastases, that is metastases that are larger than 2 mm [6]. Hence, it is important that each sentinel node is cut into 2 mm thick slices and processed in one or more cassette according to the lymph node size and embedded in paraffin wax. One H&E stained section is examined from each paraffin block. The British guidelines do not advocate cutting levels or doing immunohistochemistry with pancytokeratin. The idea is that such extra techniques, if they ever yield any metastases, these are usually in the form of isolated tumour cells, the detection of which would not alter the management of the disease. However, we occasionally examine further levels if a micrometastasis is detected, in order to exclude the possibility that the metastasis is not larger in deeper sections. Also, sentinel nodes that are less than 5 mm across are processed intact and examined at three levels. We also occasionally do immunohistochemistry for pancytokeratin (usually AE1/AE3), if the H&E section shows suspicious cells, particularly in cases of invasive lobular carcinoma, in order to exclude or confirm the presence of metastasis.

We do not routinely do frozen section examination on sentinel lymph nodes, but this is sometimes requested by surgeons in patients with clinically suspicious lymph nodes whom pre-operative diagnosis of axillary lymph nodes, either by FNA or core biopsy, was unsuccessful. If frozen sections are requested on lymph nodes, the surgeon should be made aware that there is a false negative rate of up to 25% in some published series [13]. The breast Pathologist informs the surgeon and records this in his report.

Axillary Lymph Node Clearance

Axillary lymph node clearance is carried out now much less commonly than before. It is mainly restricted to patients who had pre-operative evidence of the presence of axillary node metastasis. Clearance is also carried out on patients who underwent surgery with sentinel node biopsy that proved to be positive for metastasis. However, the need for axillary clearance in some sentinel node positive patients is being questioned. The (UK) Association of Breast Surgery and American Society of Clinical Oncology recommended omitting axillary clearance in patients with micrometastases and in selected patients with one or two positive nodes who are going to undergo conservative surgery followed by whole breast radiotherapy [14]. Occasionally we get 'axillary sampling' where only four or five nodes are removed. Some surgeons send different levels of lymph nodes separately, others only send the apical node separately or identify it with a suture.

The number of lymph nodes in the axilla varies from one person to another. It has been estimated that the average total number is 27 (range 7–58), with an average of 11 in level I (1–30), 8 (1–24) in level II (behind the pectoralis minor muscle), and 5 (1–21) in level III (infraclavicular) [15].

All the nodes in the specimen are identified by palpation, dissected and dealt with according to their size. If they are big enough to be bisected, (5 mm or more), this is done along the presumed site of their hilum, and both halves are processed in one cassette. If the nodes are too small for bisection, they are processed intact, and in this case more than one lymph node may be processed in the same cassette. If a lymph node is too big to be included in a cassette and there is obvious tumour involvement, only one slice of that node is processed. If the enlarged node does not show obvious macroscopic deposits, the whole node is sectioned horizontally and processed in two or more cassettes. The whole idea is to keep track of the number of lymph nodes dissected from the specimen. Hence, it is vital to record in the block description sheet the number of nodes in each cassette. We usually examine one H&E stained section from each paraffin block. In cases of invasive lobular carcinomas, as mentioned above, immunocyto-chemistry for pancytokeratin is carried out if suspicious atypical cells are detected in an H&E stained section.

Examination of Breast Tissue After Neo-adjuvant Chemotherapy

After confirming the diagnosis of breast carcinoma by a core biopsy and establishing its histological type, grade, ER and HER2 status, many patients with large, high grade tumours may receive 4–6 cycles of (neo-adjuvant) chemotherapy, mainly to reduce the size of the tumour before removing what is left of it, surgically.

Chemotherapy given before removing the tumour can have no effect, reduce the size of the tumour, or sometimes make it completely disappear. During the chemotherapy course, the response of the tumour is assessed by clinical and radiological examination. If there is rapid reduction in the tumour size, a 'tumour marker' is inserted by the Radiologist, during follow-up radiography, to facilitate later surgery. This also helps identifying the site of the tumour by the Pathologist particularly in cases where there is pathological complete response. The factors associated with such complete response include HER2 positivity, ER negativity [16] and the presence of high levels of tumour infiltrating lymphocytes (TILs) [17]. Ductal carcinoma is more likely to respond than lobular, although we have seen pathological complete response in cases of HER2 positive pleomorphic lobular carcinoma (unpublished observation).

The specimens received after neo-adjuvant chemotherapy could be in the form of a wire localization biopsy, a wide local excision or a mastectomy. These can be associated with sentinel lymph node biopsy or an axillary node clearance. Processing the specimen will depend on whether there is or there is no obvious residual tumour in the specimen. If there is an obvious tumour, the specimen is dealt with in the usual way as described above. If there is no obvious tumour, every effort should be made to identify the original site of the tumour, and thoroughly sample the area. If there are lymph nodes, all have to be processed and examined thoroughly for the presence of metastasis or chemotherapy changes. It is important to establish whether there is any residual tumour or not as pathological complete response is thought to be an indication of better patient outcome and that the outcome correlates with the pathological nodal status [18].

Steps of Gross Examination

1. **If there is an obvious tumour**
   The specimen is dealt with as explained in the previous sections.
2. **If there is no obvious tumour, and there is a marker**
   Identify the marker in the specimen: this usually can be seen during slicing the specimen. If the marker is not identified during dissection, specimen x-ray may have to be carried out to localize it (Fig. 6.10)
   Remove the marker and process all tissue around it

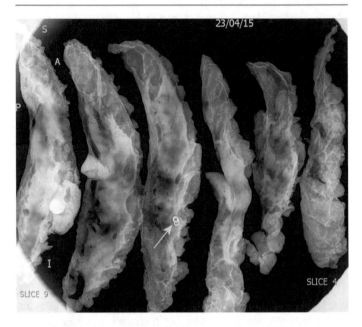

Fig. 6.10 X-ray of mastectomy slices from a patient who had neoadjuvant chemotherapy identifying the marker in slice 7 (arrow). There is no identifiable tumour. Tissue will be selected for examination from around the marker in slice 7 as well as from the corresponding areas in slices 6 and 8

+ Any other suspicious areas

+ All lymph nodes: These may be particularly difficult to detect, because of fibrosis and reduction in size

3. **If there is no obvious tumour and no marker**

   In mastectomy specimens: it is essential to know beforehand, which quadrant or area the tumour was. The site of the tumour may be identified, grossly, as a fibrotic stellate area that looks different from surrounding tissue. This area has to be sampled thoroughly (as well any other suspicious areas)

   In wide local excisions: A specimen of a reasonable size (say up to 40 g) should be sliced and processed in its entirety. For larger specimens, all fibrotic areas have to be processed as well as all margins.

References

1. Rageth CJ, O'Flynn EA, Pinker K, et al. Second International Consensus Conference on lesions of uncertain potential in the breast (B3 lesions). Breast Cancer Res Treat. 2019;174:279–96.
2. Dash I, Dessauvagie B, Hardie M, et al. Mucocele-like lesions: is surgical excision still necessary? Clin Radiol. 2017;72(11):992e1–6.
3. Abraham SC, Fox K, Fraker D, Solin L, Reynolds C. Sampling of grossly benign breast reexcisions. A multidisciplinary approach to assessing adequacy. Am J Surg Pathol. 1999;23:316–22.
4. Holland R, Connolly JL, Gelman R, et al. The presence of an extensive intraductal component following a limited excision correlates with prominent residual disease in the remainder of the breast. J Clin Oncol. 1990;8:113–8.
5. Schnitt SJ, Wang HH. Histologic sampling of grossly benign breast biopsies. How much is enough? Am J Surg Pathol. 1989;13:505–12.
6. Magire A, Brogi E. Sentinel lymph nodes for breast carcinoma: an update on current practice. Histopathology. 2016;68:152–67.
7. Schwartz GF, Giuliano AE, Veronesi U, the Consensus Conference Committee. Proceedings of the Consensus Conference on the role of sentinel lymph node biopsy in carcinoma of the breast April 19 to 22, 2001, Philadelphia, Pennsylvania. Hum Pathol. 2002;33:579–89.
8. Cochran AJ. Surgical pathology remains pivotal in the evaluation of 'sentinel' lymph nodes. Am J Surg Pathol. 1999;23:1169–72.
9. Cohen LF, Breslin TM, Kuerer HM, Ross MI, Hunt KK, Sahin AA. Identification and evaluation of axillary sentinel lymph nodes in patients with breast carcinoma treated with neoadjuvant chemotherapy. Am J Surg Pathol. 2000;24:1266–72.
10. Fitzgibbons PL, LiVolsi VA, the Surgical Pathology Committee of the College of American Pathologists, the Association of Directors of Anatomic and Surgical Pathology. Recommendation for handling radioactive specimens obtained by sentinel lymphadenectomy. Am J Surg Pathol. 2000;24:1549–51.
11. Ranshaw AA, Kish R, Gould EW. Increasing radiation from sentinel node specimens in pathology over time. Am J Clin Pathol. 2010;134:299–302.
12. McMasters KM, Tuttle TM, Carlson DJ, Brown CM, Noyes RD, Glaser RL, Vennekotter DJ, Turk PS, Tate PS, Sardi A, Pb C, Edwards MJ. Sentinel lymph node biopsy for breast cancer: a suitable alternative to routine axillary dissection in multi-institutional practice when optimal technique is used. J Clin Oncol. 2000;18:2560–6.
13. Dixon JM, Mamman U, Thomas J. Accuracy of intraoperative frozen-section analysis of axillary lymph nodes. Br J Surg. 1999;86:392–5.
14. Lyman GH, Tamin S, Edge SB, Newman LA, Turner RR, Weaver DI, et al. Sentinel lymph node biopsy for patients with early stage breast can-

cer. American Society of Clinical Oncology clinical practice guideline update. J Clin Oncol. 2014;32:1365–83.

15. Cserni G. How to improve low lymph node recovery rates from axillary clearance specimens of breast cancer: a short term audit. J Clin Pathol. 1998;51:846–9.

16. Derks MGM, van de Velde CJH. Neoadjuvant chemotherapy in breast cancer: more than just downsizing. Lancet Oncol. 2018;19:2–3.

17. Denkert C, Loibe S, Noske A, et al. Tumor-associated lymphocytes as an independent predictor of response to neoadjuvant chemotherapy in breast cancer. J Clin Oncol. 2010;28:105–13.

18. Crtazar P, Zhang L, Untch M, et al. Pathological complete response and long-term clinical benefit in breast cancer: the CTNeoBC pooled analysis. Lancet. 2014;384:164–72.

Reporting Excised Cancer Specimens

7

Introduction

This is the final step in reporting breast biopsies and entails microscopic examination of sections of the selected parts of the specimen, interpreting the findings and concludes by providing a final diagnosis

It is advisable that the same pathologist who has dealt with the gross specimen and sampled it does the microscopic reporting. Gross examination, as well as clinical information, can provide the pathologist with a good idea about what to expect on microscopic examination. Even a good gross description cannot replace seeing the actual lesion by the naked eye (Fig. 7.1). However, this might not be possible in busy laboratories, but if dissection or 'grossing' is going to be carried out by a Trainee or a Pathologist Assistant, the reporting Pathologist should play an active role in supervising the process particularly in identifying the tumour and its relationship to the excision margins, especially if the patient has had neo-adjuvant chemotherapy.

A written report should, ideally, provide clear answers to a number of specific questions including the nature of the lesion and whether it is benign or malignant, and if malignant is it in situ or invasive, its histological type, size and degree of differentiation, the presence or absence of lympho-vascular invasion, calcification, necrosis and lymphocytic infiltration. In carcinomas a

© Springer Nature Switzerland AG 2020
S. Shousha, *Breast Pathology in Clinical Practice*, In Clinical Practice, https://doi.org/10.1007/978-3-030-42386-5_7

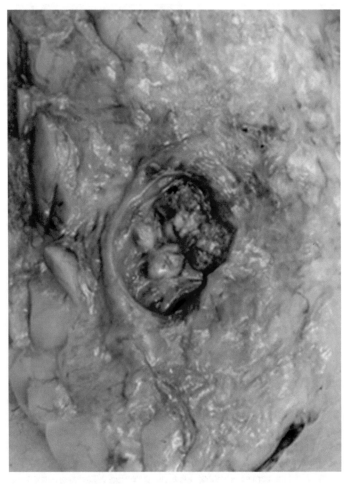

Fig. 7.1 Gross appearance of an intracystic papillary carcinoma

statement of the receptor status should be added, which can be obtained in most cases from the core biopsy report. If lymph nodes were provided their total number and the number of involved nodes is stated. Finally, the pathological stage of the tumour should be mentioned. Most of these items have been extensively discussed in the chapters dealing with reporting core biopsies. We will concentrate in this chapter on the additional items that are specifically related to the excised tumour.

Un-expected Invasive Carcinoma, Micro-invasion and Pseudo-Invasion

Un-expected invasive focus or foci, more than 1 mm in size, are sometimes seen in specimens resected for DCIS, most commonly in association with extensive high grade DCIS (Fig. 7.2). These should be measured and stated in the report. If multiple, they all usually have similar morphology. The largest focus should be chosen to carry out receptor and HER2 assessment.

Microinvasion is defined as the presence of one or more foci of clearly invasive carcinoma, none more than 1 mm across, in the immediate vicinity of duct(s) involved by ductal carcinoma in

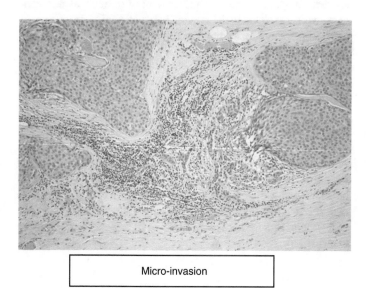

Micro-invasion

Fig. 7.2 Unexpected focus of micro-invasive carcinoma associated with foci of high grade DCIS, on either side. The invasive elements are heavily infiltrated with lymphocytes

situ [1]. A section with one of these foci should be selected for receptor and HER2 assessment.

In this respect, care should be taken not to include tumour cells displaced in the stroma, as a result of previous needling procedures, as true invasion [2]. In these cases of pseudo-invasion, the trauma of the procedure, in the form of localised haemorrhage, cholesterol crystals or track fibrosis, are always evident nearby and admixed with the dislodged tumour cells (Fig. 7.3). This process is more commonly noted after core biopsies of papillary lesions.

In general, microinvasion is not common, and tends to be seen more in association with high grade, HER2 positive cases [3], although it is sometimes seen in association with lower grades DCIS as well as in cases of LCIS. In two series from the same American Institute, displacement was more common with 14-gauge (28%) than with 11-gauge (7%) needles [2, 4]. In another study, the incidence and amount of tumour displacement was inversely related to the interval between core biopsy and excision, suggesting that tumour cells probably do not survive displacement [5].

DCIS in Association with Invasive Carcinoma

The presence or absence of DCIS elements within or adjacent to the invasive tumour should be mentioned in the report. The grade of DCIS and its extent are recorded. If DCIS is extending for a distance beyond the invasive tumour, this distance should be measured and how far this is from the excision margin is determined (Fig. 7.4). It has been noted that invasive tumours with extensive DCIS are more likely to have positive margins on excision [6].

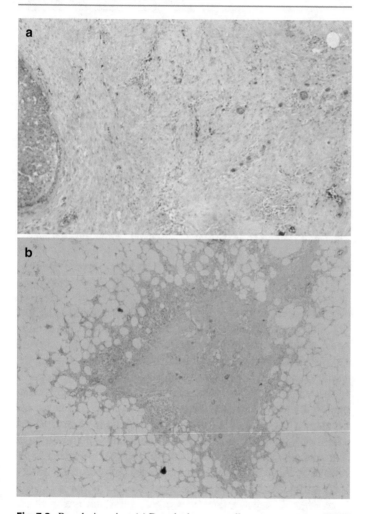

Fig. 7.3 Pseudo-invasion. (**a**) Detached tumour cells are present near a DCIS focus embedded in fibrous tissue and associated with inflammatory cells. (**b**) A focus of pseudo-invasion within fibrous needle tract surrounded by inflammatory cells and fat necrosis

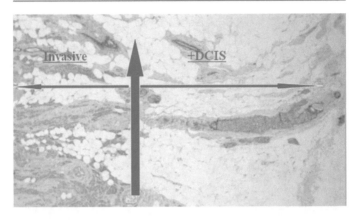

Fig. 7.4   Measuring DCIS elements present beyond the invasive tumour

Tumour Size

Accurate measurement is important for staging the disease and planning postoperative treatment. The largest dimension is measured during gross examination. For small tumours, where a cross section of the whole lesion can be included in a single slide, microscopic measurement is usually more accurate than gross measurement. In the presence of abundant DCIS elements adjacent to the invasive lesion, these are characterised and measured separately. Cases of pure DCIS can be difficult to measure if the extent of the lesion is not grossly obvious and is found in more than one microscopic section. In these cases, an assessment may have to be made on the basis of the number of consecutive slices involved by the tumour and the approximate thickness of each slice. Thus, if 3 consecutive slices, each 5 mm-thick, are involved; the estimated maximum dimension would be 15 mm, if that is more than the measurement of the lesion in individual slides.

In many cases the microscopic measurement is larger than the radiologic measurement. Thus in invasive tumours, 'tails' of tumour tissue may extend beyond the main bulk of the tumour noted radiologically. In DCIS, particularly when the radiologic assessment relied on the presence of microcalcification, DCIS foci with no microcalcification may extend beyond those with calcium.

For TNM classification, only the size of the invasive tumour is considered. However, the extent of DCIS outside the invasive tumour has to be mentioned in the report. This can be useful if the radiologic and microscopic sizes need to be compared. Intracystic and solid papillary carcinomas are considered in situ lesions. When these are associated with an invasive focus, only the size of that focus is considered for TNM classification.

Complete Removal of Lesions by Core/Vacuum Biopsy

With the introduction of wider needles for core biopsies, lesions may be removed in their entirety by this procedure [7–9]. Thus, in a study of 51 cases of invasive carcinomas using stereotactic 11-gauge directional vacuum-assisted biopsy followed by surgical excision, no residual carcinoma was detected in 10 cases (20%). Complete excision was more likely to occur if 14 cores or more were taken. In these cases, tumour size can be assessed either from the imaging studies done before the biopsy, or by measuring the tumour microscopically in the core biopsy. The latter measurement tends to underestimate the maximum dimension of the tumour [7]. In another study of 667 benign lesions, complete removal was suggested by follow up mammography in 9% of lesions for which 14-gauge needles were used, and in 64% of lesions for which 11-gauge vacuum-assisted biopsy technique was employed [8]. For this reason, it is usually useful to place a localising device, like a metal clip at the site of the biopsy after taking the cores, to facilitate accurate localisation of the lesion's site if subsequent surgical excision is expected to be carried out.

Presence or Absence of Lympho-Vascular Invasion

This is usually assessed in the breast tissue just outside the tumour. The idea is to avoid confusing shrinkage artefacts, which may occur within the tumour because of poor fixation, with lymphatic

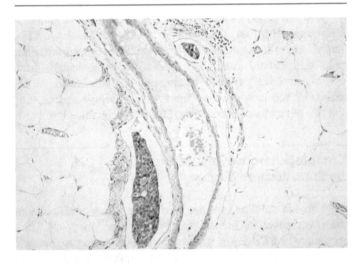

Fig. 7.5 Lympho-vascular invasion. In this case, tumour emboli are present within thin-walled vascular spaces, most likely lymphatics, on either side of a vein

invasion. The tumour cells should be present within an endothelium-lined vessel. These can usually be identified in routine H&E stained sections, without the need for special immunostaining with endothelial markers (Fig. 7.5). Distinction between lymphatics and capillaries can be difficult, hence the use of the term 'lympho-vascular' to cover both types of vessels. In many cases the involved vessel is present in the immediate vicinity of a vein and/or an artery, which helps to confirm its 'lympho-vascular' nature.

There is a good direct correlation between the presence of lympho-vascular invasion and the presence of lymph node metastasis [10], but cases with lympho-vascular invasion and no obvious lymph node metastasis do exist; and it has been shown that there is a significant relationship between lympho-vascular invasion and both survival and local recurrence, which is independent of the lymph node status [11]. Although it sounds illogical to report the absence of lympho-vascular invasion in the presence of documented lymph node metastasis, this has been recommended to be done as it might indicate the limited amount of lymphovascular invasion present in the lesion.

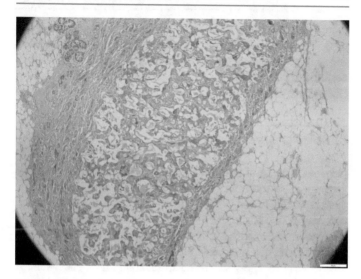

Fig. 7.6 The site of a previous vacuum biopsy including foreign body giamt cell reaction and fibrosis

Presence of Changes Indicating the Site of Previous Core/Vacuum Biopsy

The site of a previous core or vacuum biopsy can usually be identified in the sections by the presence of a localised area of fat necrosis, foreign body giant cell reaction, hemosiderin deposition, inflammation and fibrosis (Fig. 7.6). The extent of these changes depends on the size of the needle biopsy used. It is important to identify these areas and document its presence in the report particularly in cases where the tumour has been completely removed by the needling procedure.

Presence of Necrosis, Fibrosis, Elstosis, Microcalcification and Lymphocytic Infiltration

These if present should be mentioned in the report. Extensive necrosis is usually an indication of aggressiveness and is seen in poorly differentiated tumours, while elastosis and microcalcification are more commonly seen in well differentiated tumours. The site of calcification, whether it is in the invasive or in situ elements should be stated. Assessment of tumour infiltrating lymphocytes (LIMs) is useful in triple negative and HER2 positive breast carcinomas, as discussed in Chap. 5.

Multifocal Breast Carcinomas

Originally, the term multifocal breast carcinomas referred to the presence of two or more separate invasive tumours in the same quadrant of the breast, while the term multicenteric referred to the presence of two or more separate invasive carcinomas occupying more than one quadrant of the same breast. This proved to be impractical as the quadrants are divided arbitrary and it is not always easy to know where each quadrant starts and where it ends. So the term multicenteric has been dropped and multifocal disease is now defined as the presence of two or more macroscopically distinct lesions in the same breast simultaneously, irrespective of their location in the breast (Fig. 7.7).

Multifocality is usually evident radiologically and is confirmed by macroscopic examination particularly when the foci are away from each other. However, in some cases where the two, or more, foci are radiologically close but separate, microscopic, and even sometime macroscopic, examination detect the presence of connections between the close foci that were not obvious radiologically, and the disease in such a case should not be considered multifocal. Also the presence of small satellite foci close to the main lesion does not indicate multifocality (Fig. 7.7b). These satellite foci should be considered part of the main lesion and included in the tumour measurement. In general, to consider the tumours to be multifocal, normal tissue should be present between the foci in all sections examined. On the other hand, the presence of multiple foci of invasive carcinoma in cases of extensive DCIS is considered multifocal disease (Fig. 7.7c).

For TNM purposes, only the size of the largest invasive focus is considered, but the letter 'm' should be added to the equation, as discussed below, to indicate the presence of other smaller foci.

a TNM classification

- Use the size of the largest tumour

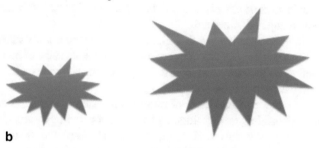

b

Satellite lesions: Small foci very close to a main lesion with no normal structures separating them

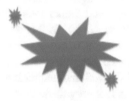

Considered part of the same lesion

c

Extensive DCIS with multiple foci of invasive carcinoma

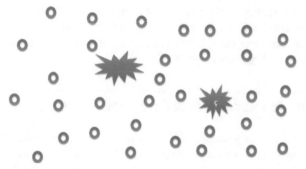

Multifocal, Use the size of the largest focus for TNM (Histology is usually the same)

Fig. 7.7 Multifocality. (**a**) Two separate foci of multifocal tumours. (**b**) Satellite foci are considered part of the main tumour. (**c**) Extensive DCIS with multifocal invasive carcinoma

It must be added here that some Oncologists insist on knowing the total tumour burden for future management, hence the report should include the sizes of all invasive foci detected no matter how many and how small.

In general patients with multifocal tumours are usually treated by mastectomy, but this depends on the number and size of foci as well as on the size of the breast. In appropriate situations, conservative surgery can be feasible [12].

The reported incidence of multifocality varies between 6 and 60% depending on definition and method of pathologic sampling. In a large study from Houston (total 3924 cases) the incidence was 24% [13]. Multifocality is more commonly seen in tumours with higher T2 stage (26% vs. 21%), show higher incidence of grade 3 (44% vs. 38%), higher incidence of lympho-vascular invasion (26% vs. 19%) and higher incidence of axillary lymph node metastasis (43% vs. 27%). In that study multicentric, (but not multifocal) tumours had worse 5 years recurrence free survival (90% vs. 95%) and 5 years survival (95% vs. 97%). However, multivariate analysis showed that neither multifocality nor multicentericity are independent prognostic factors, supporting the current use of the size of the largest lesion for TNM staging.

In multifocal lesions, even when histology appears similar, molecular characteristics may be different. The further the lesions are away from each other the more likely to be genomically different, and this may pose problems for targeted therapy [14].

In addition to the main lesion, assessment of hormone receptors and HER2 status may have to be carried out on other foci if they are large enough and particularly if they are of a different grade or histological type [15].

Has the Tumour Been Completely Excised?

Currently, an invasive tumour is only considered incompletely excised if ink is seen on the tumour cells in the sections examined [16]. If the tumour does not reach the marked margin, the distances between the various margins and the invasive and in situ elements, if present, are measured and given separately (Fig. 7.4).

The type of in situ elements seen near or at the margin is important, as most surgeons will not do further re-excision if these elements are of the LCIS type. Cavity margins, tumour bed and re-excision biopsies are reported in the same way.

Studies have shown that in cases reported as inadequately excised, the chances of finding residual tumour in the re-excision biopsies are around 55% [17]. The rate of residual tumour detection increases with the increase in the number of tissue samples examined [18]. There is evidence that the presence of increasing amount of carcinoma near the margin is associated with a significantly higher incidence of local recurrence and distal metastasis in patients with invasive breast carcinoma treated with breast-conserving surgery [19]. A positive margin is associated with a 2.5 increased risk of local recurrence, compared with negative margins. The introduction of margin guidelines dramatically decreased the rate of re-excision and mastectomies (in one centre from 21% to 15%); with associated financial savings [16].

In invasive cancers, increasing the negative margin size is not associated with a significant improvement in the rate of local recurrence. However, young patients and patients with triple negative tumours may require a wider excision margin, because of a higher rate of local recurrence; although the higher risk of recurrence in these patients may be due to the biology of the tumour rather than the distance from margin [16].

In DCIS, although 10 year mortality rate is less than 1%, after conservative surgery. Local control is important because half local recurrences are invasive, with associated increased mortality risk. Multi-centric DCIS is uncommon, but the lesions may be extensive. Ninety percent of high grade lesions grow continuously, but 70% of non-high grade lesions may have a skip pattern, with uninvolved part of the affected duct measuring less than 5 mm in 82% of cases (Fig. 7.8). Hence a margin of 2 mm at least is needed in most cases, including cases associated with micro-invasion [16] (Fig. 7.9). For patients with DCIS treated by conservative surgery alone: (17–44% of patients), a 2 mm margin minimizes the risk of local recurrence in comparison with smaller margins. A margin larger than 2 mm does not seem to reduce the risk of recurrence any further. However, the grade and the size of

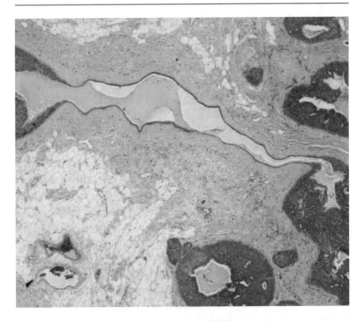

Fig. 7.8 DCIS involving parts of a duct with normal area in-between

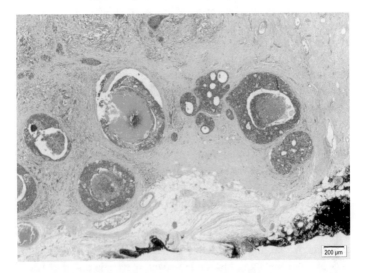

Fig. 7.9 DCIS with microinvasion, excised with less than 1 mm from inked margin. Tumour recurred within 2 years

the lesion as well as the patient's age have to be taken in consideration when deciding the appropriate margin size, which in some centres would go up to 5 mm.

Axillary Lymph Node Status

Nodes with grossly obvious metastasis are easily found and diagnosed. The maximum dimension of the largest tumour deposit in the positive node has to be given in the report. Sometimes a clinically markedly enlarged node appears microscopically as if it is the result of several amalgamated, adjacent involved nodes. We mention this possibility in the report although the 'node' is still counted as one. The presence or absence of extra-nodal tumour spread outside the lymph node capsule is mentioned, as it might have an effect on management and prognosis [20] (Fig. 7.10). For nodes with no obvious gross involvement, sections are scanned by the low power

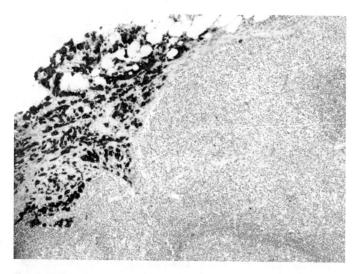

Fig. 7.10 Extra-capsular tumour spread. The metastatic carcinoma extends beyond the lymph node capsule into adjacent fatty tissue (Immunohistochemistry, AE1/AE3)

of the microscope, before going to the high power, looking care-fully for evidence of metastatic disease. We do not routinely use cytokeratin staining for the detection of micrometastasis or isolated tumour cells, as this would be impractical when dealing with an average of 20 nodes from each case and in most cases their detection will not change the management of the disease [21]. However, we sometime use cytokeratin staining in cases of invasive lobular carcinoma to confirm the malignant nature of suspicious cells.

Isolated tumor cells are defined as a small cluster of cells less than 0.2 mm, or scattered tumour cells less than 200, identified in a single section stained by H&E or cytokeratin immunohisto-chemistry (IHC) (Fig. 7.11). Tumour cells identified in different cross sections or levels cut of the same node, are not added together. Micrometastases are defined as a focus or multiple foci each more than 0.2 mm or more than 200 tumour cells, but less than 2 mm (Fig. 7.12). Extra-capsular tumour spread is defined as the presence of tumour cells within the fibrofatty tissue outside the fibrous capsule of the lymph node (Fig. 7.10).

Benign Epithelial Inclusions in Axillary Lymph Nodes

Rarely, keratin-positive benign epithelial inclusions are found in axillary nodes. It seems that they are now increasingly seen in senti-nel node biopsies, and can be mistaken for metastatic carcinoma [21]. However, in most cases they can be distinguished from carci-noma, by the lack of malignant cytological and histological features.

Four types have been described [22, 23]

1. Glandular breast like inclusions: Myoepithelial cells are pres-ent around the glands. Negative for WT1. Can show all patho-logical changes that can be seen in the breast (Fig. 7.13)
2. Glandular Mullerian like inclusions (nodal endosalpingiosis): Myoepithelial cells absent. Cells are ciliated and are WT1 pos-itive.
3. Squamous inclusions: solid or cystic.
4. Mixed glandular and squamous inclusions

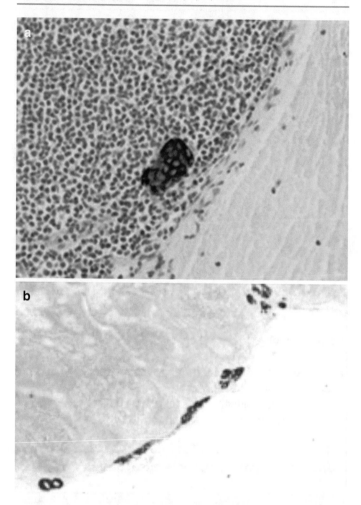

Fig. 7.11 Isolated tumour cells in lymph node. (**a**) Small cluster less than 0.2 mm. (**b**) Scattered tumour cells, less than 200 (IHC, AE1/AE3)

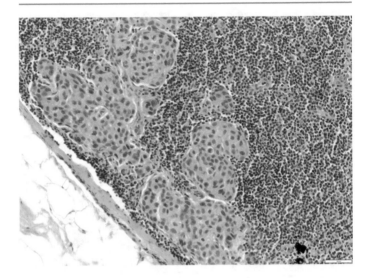

Fig. 7.12 Micrometastasis measuring 1 mm in a lymph node, seen easily in H&E stained section

Possible aetiology:

1. Transported epithelium from the breast (possibly in some cases that had breast surgery)
2. Embryologic epithelial nests (as sometimes seen with no previous breast surgery)

Additional Immunohistochemical Stains

As immunohistochemistry for ER, PR, HER2 and sometimes E-Cadherin and other markers that are needed for making a diagnosis are carried out on the core biopsy, there is usually no need to carry out additional tests on the excised tumour. The exceptions would be assessing the receptors and HER2 status for any other tumours detected, and occasionally pancytokeratin staining of a lymph node or nodes suspected of harbouring metastasis in cases of invasive lobular carcinoma.

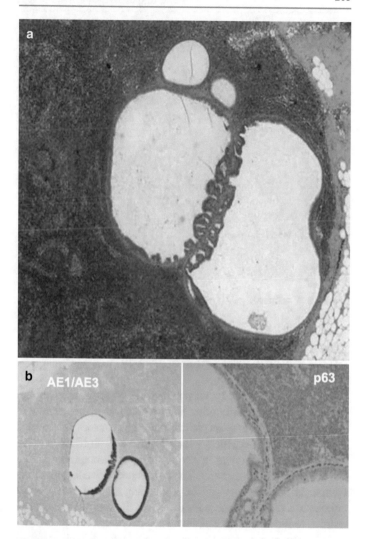

Fig. 7.13 Benign Breast-like glandular inclusions within an axillary lymph node. (**a**) H&E. (**b**) (Left) Inclusions are positive for AE1/AE3. (Right) surrounded by myoepithelial cells positive for p63. (**c**) Inclusions negative for WT1

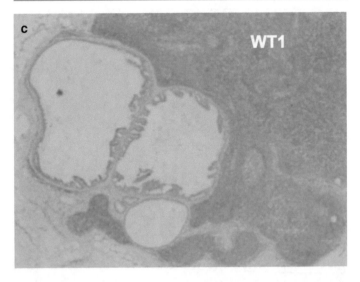

Fig. 7.13 (continued)

Reporting Excised Breast Carcinoma After Neo-adjuvant Chemotherapy

As the factors associated with pathological complete response are becoming clear, administration of neo-adjuvant chemotherapy is becoming restricted to those patients who are expected to show such a good response. These mainly include patients with HER2 positive and triple negative tumours, in whom pathological complete response has exceeded 80% in some studies [24]. Hence, the main task of the Pathologist has now changed from sampling a tumor or a residual tumour, to a thorough search for the site of the vanishing tumour in order to confirm the presence of pathological complete response.

It is uncommon now to give neo-adjuvant chemotherapy to patients with Luminal A (ER positive, HER2 negative) tumours as the rate of pathological complete response is extremely low, and has been estimated at 0.3% in one of the biggest studies [25]. It is also becoming uncommon to give such therapy to patients with invasive lobular carcinoma because of their reportedly low

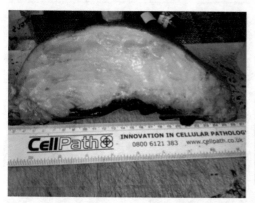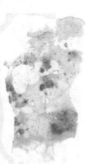

Fig. 7.14 ER positive invasive lobular carcinoma, post neoadjuvant chemotherapy, showing partial response. The gross specimen (left) shows the tumour bed as a wide area of white fibrous tissue corresponding to the actual original tumour size. H&E stained section (right) shows the presence of scattered foci of dark stained tumour cells in abundant fibrous tissue

response which has been estimated at 9% in another big study [26]. It must be added here that we have noted pathological complete response in cases of HER2 positive pleomorphic invasive lobular carcinoma (unpublished observation). Also we have noted a reasonably good, but partial, response in advanced cases of ER positive, HER2 negative classical invasive lobular carcinomas. The response in some of these cases was not obvious radiologically as there was no clear reduction in the tumour size, but was identified on microscopic examination as large parts of the remaining mass consisted of fibrous tissue (Fig. 7.14).

Gross examination should have determined whether there is a residual tumour or not, and if there is no residual tumour, the area previously occupied by the tumour has been identified and thoroughly sampled as discussed in the previous chapter.

Microscopically, the site of a disappearing tumour will be identified as an area of highly vascular fibrous tissue, devoid of any glandular structures (Fig. 7.15) and infiltrated with scattered inflammatory cells, mostly lymphocytes and foamy histiocytes. Both cellular elements may form well-defined aggregates (Fig. 7.15d). Areas of calcification may be present as well as focal

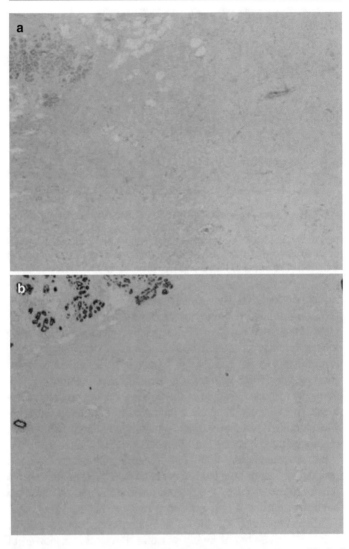

Fig. 7.15 Tumour bed in a case of pathological complete response. The bed consists of vascular fibrous tissue devoid of glandular elements. Normal glandular breast tissue is pushed at one side in this field. (**a**) H&E. (**b**) AE1/AE3. (**c**) High power view of the tumour bed with abundant blood vessels and hyalinisation. (**d**) The marker site with adjacent foreign body type multinucleated giant cells and heavy lymphocytic infiltrate

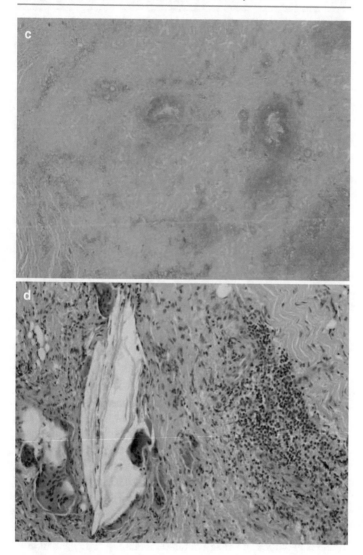

Fig. 7.15 (continued)

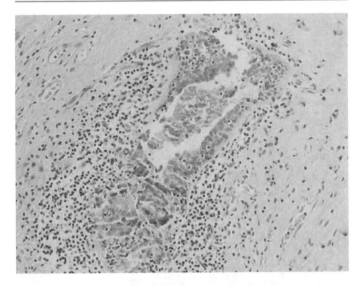

Fig. 7.16 Atypical duct heavily infiltrated with lymphocytes, present near the tumour bed

stromal mucinous change and scattered hemosiderin granules [27]. An occasional residual focus of DCIS may be present, but this is not against a diagnosis of pathological complete response. The adjacent normal glandular breast elements are sometimes clearly seen pushed at one side of this area of fibrosis (Fig. 7.15), with some of the ducts being heavily infiltrated with lymphocytes (Fig. 7.16). The rest of the breast may show ductal dilation, microcalcification and areas of sclerosing adenosis. The amount and extent of these changes vary from one case to another and sometimes can be seen in more than one area of the specimen if the patient had multiple tumours. We used to do PanCytokeratin immunohistochemistry for some of these cases as sometimes histiocytes may look like residual tumour cells Fig. 7.17) and tumour cells may look like histiocytes (Fig. 7.18). We hardly ever do that nowadays after gaining experience of what actual residual tumour cells look like with their usually dark stained pleomorphic nuclei.

As the rate of pathological complete response is increasing, there are currently Trials trying to find out if surgery can be

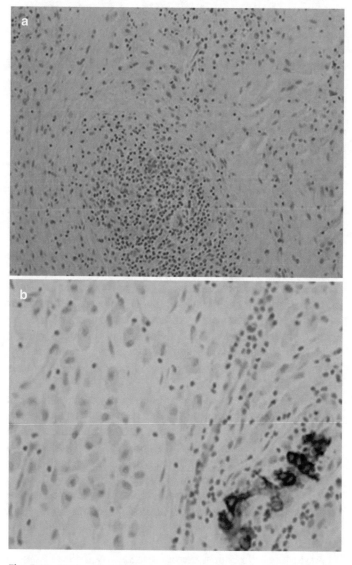

Fig. 7.17 Histiocytic infiltration after neoadjuvant chemotherapy, looking like tumour cells. (**a**) H&E (also note the presence of a lymphocytic aggregate). (**b**) The cells are AE1/AE3 negative, seen here adjacent to a normal duct

avoided in patients with radiological evidence of complete response. For that purpose fine needle aspiration and core biopsies are taken from different parts of the tumour bed for microscopic examination and the results compared with those obtained by later surgery. Pathological complete response has been correctly diagnosed in 97% of cases using a combination of ultrasound guided fine needle aspiration and vacuum assisted core biopsy [28], suggesting that in the future surgery might become safely avoided in some of these patients.

If there is residual invasive carcinoma in the excised specimen, this may be in the form of a few scattered tumour cells, singly or in small groups or could be in the form of large solid groups separated by variable amount of fibrous tissue. Much less commonly, the residual tumour is in the form of a single mass (Fig. 7.14). The residual tumour cells usually show marked nuclear pleomorphism, but little or no mitotic activity. Hence the tumour grade may sometimes change from an original grade 3 down to grade 2. The presence of scanty scattered tumour cells may simulate invasive lobular carcinoma (Fig. 7.18), but E-Cadherin, if the tumour was originally positive, stays positive. Giant tumour cells may be seen and occasionally intracellular mucin becomes evident (Fig. 7.19). The presence of lymphovascular invasion after neoadjuvant chemotherapy is strongly associated with poor prognosis and local relapse [29].

Chemotherapy may change the hormone receptor and hER2 status of residual tumour as well as other markers in a minority of cases. In a limited study of 25 cases: ER remained the same in 80%, up in 12%, down in 8% PR: same in 80%, up in 8%, down in 12% and HER2: same in 80%, up in 12%, down in 8%, ki67: same in 76%, up in 4%, down in 20% p53: same in 96%, up in 4%, down in 0 [30]. In practice we do not re-assess the receptor status on any residual tumour. However, in cases of recurrences it is advisable to repeat the tests on the recurrent tumour if obtaining a tissue sample is feasible.

Assessment of residual tumour size is easy if thee is only a single focus remaining (Fig. 7.20). If there are several residual foci in place of an original single tumour, the overall maximum dimension of the area occupied by the scattered foci has to be

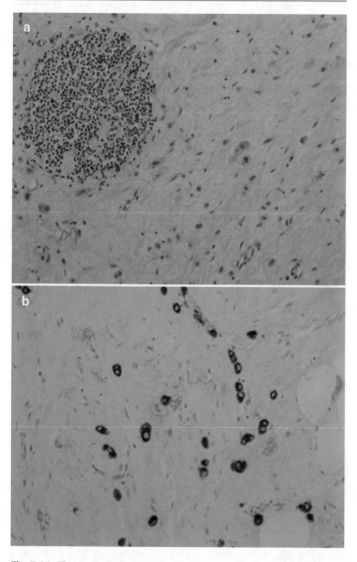

Fig. 7.18 Tumour cells looking like histiocytes in H&E stained section (**a**), but are strongly positive for AE1/AE3 (**b**). Note also that the cells are arranged in a lobular pattern, although the tumour is of a ductal phenotype

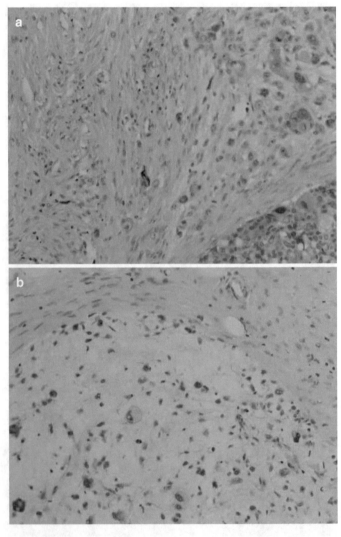

Fig. 7.19 Change in morphology after chemotherapy. (**a**) Part of the tumour is solid and part is in the form of scattered tumour cells in a fibrous stroma, including multi-nucleated giant tumour cells. (**b**) Tumour cells scattered in a mucinous stroma. (**c**) Tumour cells forming well-differentiated mucin containing glandular structures

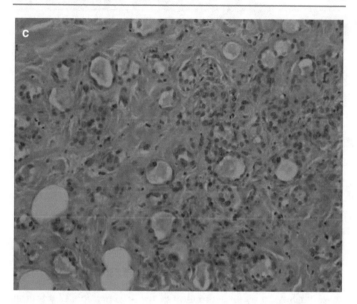

Fig. 7.19 (continued)

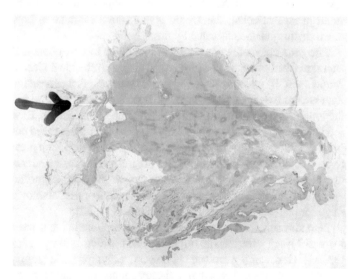

Fig. 7.20 A single focus of residual invasive tumour, beside the site of a marker on the left hand side (arrow)

Assessment of residual tumour size

☐ Easy if there is a residual single focus

☐ Difficult when there are several residual foci:
    ☐ But as they are presumably all parts of the original tumour, the overall maximum dimension of the area occupied by the scattered foci has to be given.
    ☐ An estimation of the area occupied by tumour (say 20% in this example) may be added

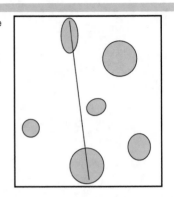

Fig. 7.21 Assessment of residual tumour size after neo-adjuvant chemotherapy

given, followed by an estimation of the area occupied by tumour cells (say 20%) (Fig. 7.21). The same procedure can be used if the residual tumour is in the form of a few scattered single cells or small groups of cells. This would give a rough estimate of how much the tumour was affected by the therapy.

The percentage of residual tumour in relation to the tumour bed area described above is used for calculating the 'Residual Cancer Burden' (RCB) which is a scoring system based on that percentage figure as well as the number of residually positive lymph nodes, and the longest diameter of the largest residual nodal metastasis. Raw scores are then categorized into RCB classes using pre-defined cut points, with a score of 0 representing pathological complete response and scores 1–3 representing progressively greater extents of residual cancer. RCB has been shown to provide prognostic value of all breast cancer phenotypes, independent of the pathologic stage for patients with stage II and III disease [31, 32].

Neoadjuvant chemotherapy eradicates lymph node metastases in up to 74% of patients who originally had positive axillary nodes [33, 34]. Hence, it is advocated to do sentinel lymph node biopsy, at the time of surgical excision in these patients, to avoid carrying out unnecessary axillary node clearance.

In general, microscopic examination of available axillary Lymph Nodes can show one of three possible features:

1. They may appear normal/reactive, if they were not previously involved by metastasis.
2. They may show evidence of 'Tumour regression' which may take various forms, the most common being wide areas of fibrosis which may be hyalinised and associated with foamy histiocytes and sometimes haemosidren deposits. Less common is the presence of pure large accumulations of foamy histiocytes. Mucin pools and areas of microcalcification may be also present (Fig. 7.22). The areas showing these changes are supposed to be the areas that were occupied by metastasis. Sometimes a few residual tumour cells are seen in these areas, if so, the node should be considered positive for metastasis. Occasionally a pancytokeratin immunohistochemistry may be indicated if there are suspicious cells within the 'regressed' areas to find out whether they are malignant epithelial cells or not (Figs. 7.23 and 7.24).
3. The lymph node may show metastasis with no evidence of tumour regression.

Patients with axillary lymph nodes showing evidence of tumour regression have intermediate prognosis between those with residual lymph node metastasis and those with negative nodes [35].

Gene Expression Profiling

Patients with ER positive breast carcinoma are usually treated with adjuvant endocrine therapy, in addition to surgery. The addition of adjuvant chemotherapy can reduce the recurrence risk by 25–30%. Gene expression profiling helps deciding which patients would benefit from having chemotherapy and those who would not benefit and therefore can avoid the side effects associated with chemotherapy. The test can be done on core biopsies as well as on excised tumours using routinely processed formalin fixed, paraffin embedded tumour tissue.

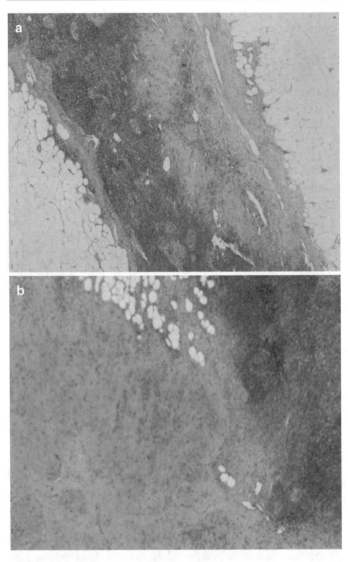

Fig. 7.22 Lymph nodes showing post neoadjuvant chemotherapy changes. (**a**) Hilar fibrosis. (**b**) Extensive hyalinised fibrous tissue. (**c**) Extensive infiltration with foamy histiocytes. These are all probably the sites of completely responding metastases

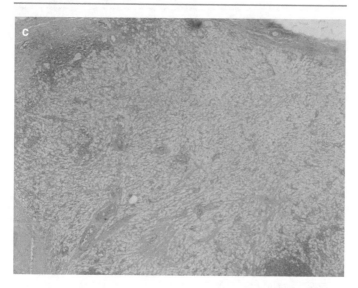

Fig. 7.22 (continued)

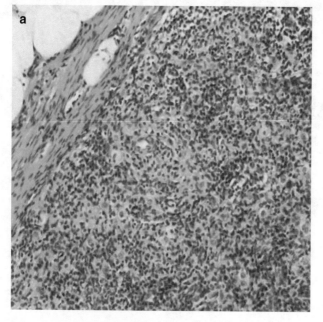

Fig. 7.23 Lymph nodes showing post neoadjuvant chemotherapy changes associated with the presence of suspicious residual tumour cells. (**a**) H&E. (**b**) AE1/AE3

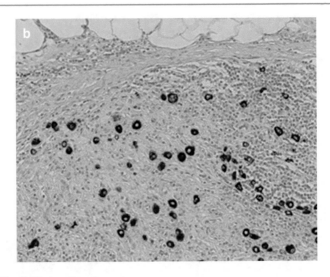

Fig. 7.23 (continued)

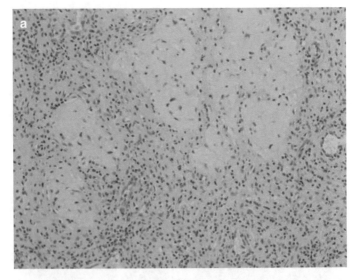

Fig. 7.24 Lymph node showing post neoadjuvant chemotherapy change in the form of mucinous areas containing suspicious cells (**a**) that proved to be scattered AE1/AE3 positive tumour cells (**b**)

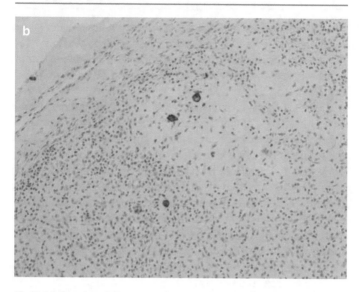

Fig. 7.24 (continued)

The role of Histopathologists in these procedures is usually limited to selecting the appropriate paraffin block with enough representative tumour tissue to carry out the test. In cases of multifocal tumours with different grades or morphology, a paraffin block representing each tumour may be selected. The test in these cases is done first on the tumour that is more likely to be most aggressive, for example a grade 3 tumour rather than a grade 1 or 2. If the recurrence score is high, indicating a need for chemotherapy, there is no need to do the test on the other tumours. Several tests are available, the two commonly used are Oncotype DX and EndoPredict.

Oncotype DX® (Genomic Health, Redwood city, California) is a 21-gene expression assay that estimates the risk of recurrence and benefit from adjuvant chemotherapy for patients with ER positive, HER2 negative breast cancer. This is a reverse transcriptase polymerase chain reaction based on assessing genes associated with tumour invasion and proliferation and including, among others, ER, PR, HER2 and Ki67. A score is calculated and patients are categorised based on a recurrence score (RS) into low, intermediate and high risk of distant recurrence, with the latter group being the one most likely in need of having chemotherapy . The RS has been validated for predicting benefit from chemotherapy using retrospective analysis of large number of ER positive, HER2 negative breast cancer cases [36].

EndoPredict® is a multi-gene test for breast cancer patients based on analysis of tumour genes in combination with the classical prognostic factors of nodal status and tumour size. It detects the likelihood of late metastases (i.e., metastasis formation after more than 5 years) and can thus guide treatment decisions for chemotherapy as well as extended anti-hormonal therapy. The test was shown to be able to predict cancer-specific disease progression and metastasis in multiple clinical outcome studies with more than 3000 patients. The test is appropriate for pre- and post-menopausal women diagnosed with ER positive, HER2 negative early stage breast cancer with either node-negative or node-positive disease (1–3 nodes) [37].

As these gene profiling tests are expensive, attempts have been made to use the much cheaper immunohistochemical tests for ER, PR, HER2 and Ki67 as well as general histopathological features to replace them or reduce the need to use them [38, 39].

Pathological Staging of Breast Carcinoma

The pathological stage of the disease should be stated at the end of the report as it is important for planning the post-operative management of the disease. Following are detailed description of the traditional staging method and a modified, simplified version of the recently suggested Pathologic prognostic staging.

The Traditional TNM Pathological Staging of Breast Carcinoma [40]

Primary tumour (pT):

- pTx. Primary tumour cannot be assessed
- pTo. No evidence of primary tumour
- pTis. (DCIS) ductal carcinoma in situ

- pTis. (Paget). Paget's disease of the nipple (not associated with DCIS)
- pT1mic. Invasive tumour 1 mm or less (microinvasive). Multiple microinvasive foci are not added together.
- pT1a. Tumour larger than 1 mm and not more than 5 mm
- pT1b. Tumour larger than 5 mm and not more than 10 mm
- pT1c. Tumour larger than 10 mm and not more than 20 mm
- pT2. Tumour larger than 20 mm and not more than 50 mm
- pT3. Tumour more than 50 mm in largest dimension
- pT4a. Tumour of any size extending to chest wall (not only pectoralis muscle)
- pT4b. Tumour of any size with direct extension to the skin causing ulceration and/or skin satellite nodules and/or skin oedema or peau d'orange involving less than one third of the skin (invasion of the dermis alone does not qualify for pT4)
- pT4c. Tumour of any size extending to both chest wall and skin
- pT4d. Inflammatory carcinoma, which is characterised by the presence of diffuse oedema or peau d'orange involving one third or more of the breast skin.

Notes:
- m is added at the beginning of the stage if there are multiple foci of invasive tumour, but staging is based on the size of the largest tumour,
- r is added for recurrent tumours
- y is added post-neoadjuvant treatment

Axillary lymph nodes status (pN):
- pNx. Lymph nodes not available for assessment
- pN0. No metastasis or only isolated tumour cells identified. Isolated tumour cells are defined as a small cluster of cells less than 0.2 mm, or scattered tumour cells less than 200, identified in a single section stained by H&E or cytokeratin immunohistochemistry (IHC). Tumour cells identified in different cross sections or levels cut of the same node, are not added together.
- pN0 (i−). No lymph node metastasis, confirmed by IHC.
- pN0 (i+). Isolated tumour cells identified by IHC

- pN0 (mol−). No metastasis by molecular (reverse transcriptase-polymerase chain reaction, RT-PCR) analysis
- pN0 (mol+). Tumour cells detected by RT-PCR, but not seen in sections stained by H&E or IHC
- pN1mi. Lymph node containing a micrometastatic focus or multiple foci (each more than 0.2 mm or more than 200 tumour cells, but less than 2 mm)
- pN1a. Metastases in 1–3 lymph nodes with at least one metastasis more than 2 mm
- pN1b. Histologically confirmed metastasis in internal mammary node in the absence of axillary metastasis
- pN1c. Metastasis present in 1–3 axillary nodes and in internal mammary node
- pN2a. Metastases in 4–9 lymph nodes with at least one metastasis more than 2 mm
- pN3a. Metastases in 10 or more lymph nodes with at least one metastasis more than 2 mm
- pN3b Metastasis in four or more axillary nodes + positive internal mammary node
- pN3c. Histologically confirmed metastasis in ipsilateral supraclavicular node(s)

Notes:
- (sn). Added at the end of N classification indicates that only sentinel lymph nodes were evaluated. (sn) not to be used if more than six sentinel/non-sentinel nodes are examined.
- Intramammary nodes are included with axillary nodes.
- Direct extension of tumour into a node is considered a positive node
- A tumour nodule in axillary fat with a smooth contour is classified as a positive node.

Distal Metastasis (M):
- cM0 (i+). No clinical evidence of distal metastasis, but molecular or microscopic tumour cells are detected in the blood or bone marrow, or in the form of microscopic deposits less than 0.2 mm in distal organs
- pM1. Distal metastatic deposits more than 0.2 mm, confirmed histologically.

Traditional Anatomic Stage prognostic groups
- Stage 0: Tis N0 M0
- Stage IA: T1 N0 M0
- Stage IB: T0/1 N1mi, M0
- Stage IIA: T0/1 N1 M0
  T2 N0 M0
- Stage IIB: T2 N1 M0
  T3 N0 M0
- Stage IIIA: T0/1/2 N2 M0
  T3 N1/2 M0
- Stage IIIB: T4 N0/1/2 M0
- Stage IIIC: Any size tumour with metastasis in more than ten lymph nodes and no distal metastasis
- Stage IV: Any size tumour with any number of positive nodes+ distal metastasis

The Modified Pathologic Prognostic Staging

In addition to the traditional TNM staging, the eighth edition of the AJCC cancer staging manual suggested adding the grade of the tumour as well as its ER, PR and HER2 status, together with the recurrence score if available [41, 42]. Tumour grade is determined using Elston & Ellis grading system [43]. ER and PR positivity is defined as any staining of 1% or more of tumour cells. HER2 positive tumours are those scoring 3+ by immunohistochemistry in at least 10% of the tumour cells. Or, if using FISH, SISH or DISH show a HER2/CEP 17 ratio of 2 or more, or show a HER2 copy number of 6 or more regardless of the ratio [44]. Patients who had neo-adjuvant chemotherapy are not assigned a pathologic prognostic stage.

Stage 0:
- Ductal carcinoma in situ with no axillary or distal metastasis, regardless of the size or grade of lesion

Stage IV
- Tumours with distal metastasis, regardless of the size or grade of tumour, the number of positive nodes or ER, PR or HER2 status

TNM0	Grade	ER	HER2	Stage
T0/1 N0/1mi	1	+	−	IA
		+	+	IA
		−	+	1A
		−	−	1A
	2	+	−	IA
		+	+	1A
		−	+	1A
		−	−	IB[a]
	3	+	−	1A
		+	+	IA
		−	+	IA
		−	−	IB[a]

[a]In the rare cases where PR is positive (ER negative), the stage is IA

TNM0	Grade	ER	HER2	Stage
T0/1 N1 and T2 N0	1	+	−	IA[a]
		+	+	IA[a]
		−	+	1B[b]
		−	−	IIA[c]
	2	+	−	IA
		+	+	1A[a]
		−	+	1B[b]
		−	−	IIA
	3	+	−	1B[b]
		+	+	IA[b]
		−	+	IIA
		−	−	IIA

[a]IB If PR is negative
[b]IIA if PR is negative
[c]IB if PR is positive

TNM0	Grade	ER	HER2	Stage
T2 N1 and T3 N0	1	+	−	IA[a]
		+	+	IA[a]
		−	+	IIB
		−	−	IIB
	2	+	−	IB[a]
		+	+	1B[a]
		−	+	1IB

TNM0	Grade	ER	HER2	Stage
		−	−	IIB
	3	+	−	IIA[a]
		+	+	IB[a]
		−	+	IIB
		−	−	IIA[b]

[a]IIB if PR is negative
[b]IIIA if PR is negative

TNM0	Grade	ER	HER2	Stage
T1/2 N2 and T3 N1/2	1	+	−	IB[a]
		+	+	IB[a]
		−	+	IIIA
		−	−	IIIA
	2	+	−	IB[a]
		+	+	1B[a]
		−	+	IIIA
		−	−	IIIB[b]
	3	+	−	IIB[a]
		+	+	IIA[a]
		−	+	IIIA
		−	−	IIIA[c]

[a]IIIA if PR is negative
[b]IIIA if PR is positive
[c]IIIC if PR is negative

TNM0	Grade	ER	HER2	Stage
T4 N0/1/2 + Any T N3	1	+	−	IIIA[a]
		+	+	IIIA[a]
		−	+	IIIB
		−	−	IIIB
	2	+	−	IIIA[a]
		+	+	IIIA[a]
		−	+	IIIB
		−	−	IIIB[b]
	3	+	−	IIIB[b]
		+	+	IIIB
		−	+	IIIB
		−	−	IIIC

[a]IIIB if PR is negative
[b]IIIC If PR is negative

TNM	Grade	ER	PR	HER2	Stage
Any T/Any N/M1	Any grade	Any	Any	Any	IV

Evaluation

- In a study of 7458 breast cancer patients with 98.7 month median follow up, the anatomic prognostic staging was more accurate in predicting 5-year and disease free survival than the traditional staging method [45]. The survival rates were found to decrease with increasing prognostic stage, which was not always the case with traditional staging [45].

References

1. National Coordinating Group for Breast Screening Pathology. Pathology reporting in breast cancer screening. 2nd ed. NHSBSP Publication No. 3; 1995.
2. Youngson BJ, Liberman L, Rosen PP. Displacement of carcinomatous epithelium in surgical breast specimens following stereotaxic core biopsy. Am J Clin Pathol. 1995;103:598–602.
3. Baqai T, Shousha S. Oestrogen receptor negativity as a marker for high-grade ductal carcinoma in situ of the breast. Histopathology. 2003;42:440–7.
4. Liberman L, Vuolo M, Dershaw DD, Morris EA, Abramson AF, LaTrnta LR, Polini NM, Rosen PP. Epithelial displacement after stereotactic 11-gauge directional vacuum-assisted breast biopsy. AJR. 1999; 172:677–81.
5. Diaz LK, Wiley EL, Venta LA. Are malignant cells displaced by large-gauge needle core biopsy of the breast? AJR. 1999;173:1303–13.
6. Jimenez RE, Bongers S, Bouwman D, Segel M, Visscher DW. Clinicopathologic significance of ductal carcinoma in situ in breast core needle biopsies with invasive cancer. Am J Surg Pathol. 2000;24:123–8.
7. Liberman L, Zakowski M, Avery S, Hudis C, Morris EA, Abramson AF, LaTrenta LR, Glassman JR, Dershaw DD. Complete percutaneous excision of infiltrating carcinoma at stereotactic breast biopsy: how can tumor size be assessed? AJR. 1999;173:1315–22.
8. Jackman RJ, Marzoni FA, Nowels KW. Percutaneous removal of benign mammographic lesions: comparison of automated large-core and directional vacuum-assisted stereotactic biopsy techniques. AJR. 1998;171: 1325–30.
9. Fine RE, Israel PZ, Walker LC, Corgan KR, Greenwald LV, Berenson JE, Boyd BA, Oliver MK, McClure T, Elberfeld J. A prospective study of the

removal rate of imaged breast lesions by an 11-gauge vacuum-assisted biopsy probe system. Am J Surg. 2001;182:335–40.

10. Yiangou C, Shousha S, Sinnett HD. Primary tumour characteristics and axillary lymph node status in breast cancer. Br J Cancer. 1999;80: 1974–8.

11. Pinder SE, Ellis IO, Galea M, O'Rouke S, Blamey RW, Elston CW. Pathological prognostic factors in breast cancer. III. Vascular invasion: relationship with recurrence and survival in a large study with long-term follow-up. Histopathology. 1994;24:41–7.

12. Afaseven B, Lederer B, Blohmer JU, et al. Impact of multifocal or multicentric disease on surgery and locoregional, distant and overall survival of 6,134 breast cancer patients treated with neoadjuvant chemotherapy. Ann Surg Oncol. 2015;22:1118–27.

13. Lynch SP, Lei X, Chavez-MacGregor M, et al. Multifocality and multicentricity in breast cancer and survival outcome. Ann Oncol. 2012;23:3063–9.

14. Salgado R, Aftimos P, Sotiriou C, et al. Evolving paradigm in multifocal breast cancer. Semin Cancer Biol. 2015;31:111–8.

15. Choi Y, Kim EJ, Seol H, et al. The hormone receptor, human epidermal growth factor receptor 2, and molecular subtype status of individual tumor foci in multifocal/multicentric invasive ductal carcinoma of breast. Hum Pathol. 2012;43:48–55.

16. Pilewskie M, Morrow M. Margins in breast cancer: how much is enough. Cancer. 2018;124:1335–41.

17. Gwin JL, Eisenberg BL, Hoffman JP, Ottery FD, Boraas M, Solin LJ. Incidence of gross and microscopic carcinoma in specimens from patients with breast cancer after re-excision lumpectomy. Ann Surg. 1993;218:729–34.

18. Abraham SC, Fox K, Fraker D, Solin L, Reynolds C. Sampling of grossly benign breast reexcisions. A multidisciplinary approach to assessing adequacey. Am J Surg Pathol. 1999;23:316–22.

19. Goldstein NS, Kestin L, Vicini F. Factors associated with ipsilateral breast failure and distant metastases in patients with invasive breast carcinoma treated with breast-conserving therapy. Am J Clin Pathol. 2003;120:500–27.

20. Fisher BJ, Perera FE, Cooke AL, Opeitum A, Dar AR, Venkatesan VM, Stitt L, Radwan JS. Extracapsular axillary node extension in patients receiving adjuvant systemic therapy: an indication for radiotherapy? Int J Radiat Oncol Biol Phys. 1997;38:551–9.

21. Lyman GH, Tamin S, Edge SB, Newman LA, Turner RR, Weaver DI, et al. Sentinel lymph node biopsy for patients with early stage breast cancer. American Society of Clinical Oncology clinical practice guideline update. J Clin Oncol. 2014;32:1365–83.

22. Fellgara G, Carcangiu ML, Rosai J. Benign epithelial inclusions in axillary lymph nodes: report of 18 cases and review of the literature. Am J Surg Pathol. 2011;35:1123–33.

23. Corben AD, Nehhozina T, Garg K, Vellejo CE, Brogi E. Endosalpingiosis in axillary lymph nodes: a possible pitfall in the staging of patients with breast carcinoma. Am J Surg Pathol. 2010;34:1211–6.
24. Derks MGM, van de Velde CJH. Neoadjuvant chemotherapy in breast cancer: more than just downsizing. Lancet Oncol. 2018;19:2–3.
25. Haque W, Verma V, Hatch S, et al. Response rates and pathologic complete response by breast cancer molecular subtype following neoadjuvant chemotherapy. Breast Cancer Res Treat. 2018;120:559–67.
26. Gentile LF, Plitas G, Zabor EC, et al. Tumor biology predicts pathologic complete response to neoadjuvant chemotherapy in patients presenting with locally advanced breast cancer. Ann Surg Oncol. 2017;24:3896–902.
27. Pinder SE, Provenzano E, Earl H, Ellis IO. Laboratory handling and histology reporting of breast specimens from patients who have received neoadjuvant chemotherapy. Histopathology. 2007;50:409–17.
28. Rauch GM, Kuerer HM, Adrada B, Santiago L, Moseley T, Candelaria RP. Biopsy feasibility trial for breast cancer pathologic complete response detection after neoadjuvant chemotherapy: imaging assessment and correlation endpoints. Ann Surg Oncol. 2018;25:1953–60.
29. Hamy A-S, Lam G-T, Lass E, et al. Lymphovascular invasion after neoadjuvant chemotherapy is strongly associated with poor prognosis in breast carcinoma. Breast Cancer Res Treat. 2018;169:295–304.
30. Arens N, Bleyl U, Hildenbrand R. HER2/neu, p53, ki67, and hormone receptors do not change during neoadjuvant chemotherapy in breast cancer. Virchows Arch. 2005;446:489–96.
31. Symmans WF, Peintinger F, Hatzis C, et al. Measurement of residual breast cancer burden to predict survival after neoadjuvant chemotherapy. J Clin Oncol. 2007;25:4414–22.
32. Symmans WF, Wei C, Gould R, et al. Long-term prognostic risk after neoadjuvant chemotherapy associated with residual cancer burden and breast cancer subtype. J Clin Oncol. 2017;35:1049–60.
33. Fisher B, Brown A, Mamounas E, et al. Effect of preoperative chemotherapy on local-regional disease in women with operable breast cancer: findings from National Surgical Adjuvant Breast and Bowel Project B-18. J Clin Oncol. 1997;15:2483–93.
34. Dominci LS, Morgan Gonzalez VM, Buzdar AU. Cytologically proven axillary lymph node metastases are eradicated in patients receiving preoperative chemotherapy with concurrent Trastuzumab for HER2-positive breast cancer. Cancer. 2010;116:2884–9.
35. Newman LA, Pernick NL. Histopathologic evidence of tumor regression in the axillary lymph nodes of patients treated with preoperative chemotherapy correlates with breast cancer outcome. Ann Surg Oncol. 2003;10:734–9.
36. Lancaster J, Armstrong A, Howell S, et al. Impact of oncotype DX breast recurrence score testing on adjuvant chemotherapy use in early breast cancer: real world experience in Greater Manchester, UK. Eur J Surg Oncol. 2017;43:931–7.

37. Filipits M, Rudas M, Jakesz R, et al. A new molecular predictor of distant recurrence in ER-positive, HER2-negative breast cancer adds independent information to conventional clinical risk factors. Clin Cancer Res. 2011;17:6012–20.

38. Cuzick J, Dowsett M, Pineda S, et al. Prognostic value of a combined estrogen receptor, progesterone receptor, Ki-67, and human epidermal growth factor receptor 2 immunohistochemical score and comparison with the Genomic Health recurrence score in early breast cancer. J Clin Oncol. 2011;29:4273–8.

39. Gage MM, Mylander WC, Rosman M, Fujii T, Le Du F, Raghavendra A, et al. Combined pathologic-genomic algorithm for early-stage breast cancer improves cost-effective use of the 21-gene recurrence score assay. Ann Oncol. 2018;29:1280–5.

40. Lester SC, Rose S, Chen Y-Y, Connolly JL, de Baca ME, Fitzgibbons PL, et al. Protocol for the examination of specimens from patients with invasive carcinoma of the breast. Arch Pathol Lab Med. 2009;133:1515–38.

41. Hortobagyi GN, Connolly JL, D'Orsi C, et al. Breast. In: Amin MB, et al., editors. AJCC cancer staging manual. 8th ed. p. 589–636. https://doi.org/10.1007/978-3-319-40618-3_48.

42. Giuliano AF, Edge SB, Hortobagyi GN. Eighth edition of the AJCC Cancer staging manual: breast cancer. Ann Surg Oncol. 2018;25:1783–5.

43. Elston CW, Ellis IO. Pathological prognostic factors in breast cancer. I. The value of histological grade in breast cancer: experience from a large study with long-term follow-up. Histopathology. 1991;19:403–10.

44. Wolff A, Hammond M, Hicks D, et al. Recommendations for human epidermal growth factor receptor 2 testing in breast cancer. American Society of Clinical Oncology/College of American Pathologists clinical practice guideline update. J Clin Oncol. 2013;31:3997–4013.

45. Lee SB, Sohn G, Kim J, et al. A retrospective prognostic evaluation analysis using the 8th edition of the American Joint Committee on Cancer staging system for breast cancer. Breast Cancer Res Treat. 2018;169:257–66.

Phyllodes Tumour

These are uncommon breast tumours and represent 2.5% of fibro-epithelial lesions and less than 1% of all breast tumours [1]. The majority (60–75%) are benign. Fifteen to twenty per cent are borderline and 10–20% are malignant. Usually present as rapidly growing mass, or accelerated growth of a previously stable lesion. Usually more than 4 cm, but can be less or much more than that. Enlargement of axillary lymph nodes may be present, but lymph node metastasis are extremely rare. Patients are usually 40–50 year old, but can occur in older and younger women and adolescents or even children and rarely in men. Two elements have to be present: stromal hypercellularity, which can be focal, and leaf-like structures which are the result of protruding stromal proliferations, covered by epithelium, into clefts or cystic spaces within the lesion. Hypercellularity, on its own, can be seen in cellular fibroadenomas, and leaf-like structures, with no hypercellularity , can be present in intracanalicular fibroadenomas (Fig. 8.1). The stromal cellularity is usually more condensed underneath the epithelium, where stromal mitotic activity can be evident. The stroma may show areas of myxomatous change and pseudoangiomatous stromal hyperplasia may be present.

Phyllodes tumours are classified into benign, border line and malignant and the grading correlates with the risk of recurrence.

© Springer Nature Switzerland AG 2020
S. Shousha, *Breast Pathology in Clinical Practice*, In Clinical
Practice, https://doi.org/10.1007/978-3-030-42386-5_8

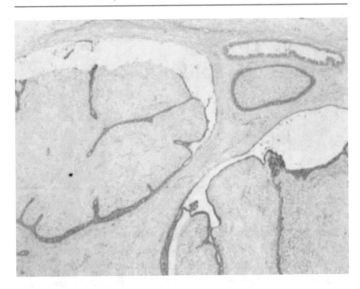

Fig. 8.1 Intra-canalicular fibroadenoma. Leaf-like structures are present but there is no stromal hypercellularity

As the morphology may vary from one area to another, the lesions must be sampled thoroughly, including areas with grossly abnormal morphology. The grade should be based on the area with the worst morphology.

Benign lesions have mild stromal hypercellularity, where the stromal nuclei are well-spaced, mild or absent nuclear atypia, less than five mitotic figures/ten HPF, absent stromal overgrowth, circumscribed pushing borders and no malignant heterologous elements. Borderline lesions have moderate stromal cellularity with mild to moderate nuclear pleomorphism, between five and nine mitotic figures, focal stromal overgrowth, circumscribed or focally infiltrative borders and no malignant heterologous elements.

Malignant lesions have marked stromal hypercellularity, with nuclei almost touching each other or overlapping, marked nuclear pleomorphism with coarse chromatin, nucleoli and irregular borders, ten or more mitotic figures, marked stromal overgrowth, infiltrative borders and may contain malignant heterologous elements, most commonly liposarcoma, but chondrosarcoma,

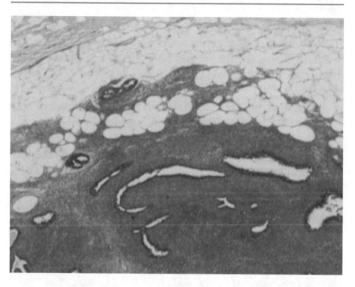

Fig. 8.2 Malignant phyllodes tumour. Note to stromal hypercellularity and the infiltrative margins

osteosarcoma, rhabdomyosarcoma or a combination of these may also occur (Fig. 8.2).

Malignant lesions have a high recurrence rate (up to 30%) and metastasis (up to 22%). The recurrence rate of benign and border-line lesions is much lower (10–17 and 14–25% respectively). Margin status is the most predictive factor for recurrence. Local recurrences usually have the same grade as the primary lesions, but could be lower or higher. Metastases usually consist of stro-mal spindle cell elements. Malignant heterologous elements may be present in the metastasis. Immunohistochemistry staining for p53, CD117, EGFR, CD10 and Ki67 may correlate with grade, but none seems to correlate with recurrence.

The stroma of phyllodes tumours, of any grade, can be positive or negative for CD34. The stroma in fibroadenomas is usually CD34 positive [2]. The stroma in both may be also positive for smooth muscle actin (myofibroblasts) [2]. The percentage of Ki-67 positively stained cells is low in benign lesions and significantly higher in low and high grade malignant lesions (3.6, 16 and 50 respectively, on average), but Ki-67 staining could not reliably predict recurrence [3]. The expression of c-myc and c-kit in the stroma is also high in malignant tumours (90% and 50% respectively), but both proteins can be expressed also in benign lesions (35% and 5% respectively) [4].

Excision of phyllodes tumour to a negative margin has been usually recommended. However, recent studies have advocated a more conservative approach for treating benign and selected borderline phyllodes without the need for re-excision if the initial excision showed a close or positive margin. This was based on the overall lower rate of recurrence (2–6%) which was not associated with the original margin status [5–7]. However, close follow up and timely excision of any recurrences are recommended.

Making a diagnosis of malignant phyllodes tumour would have serious management implications and should be taking only after thorough examination. Some authors [1] insist of making that diagnosis only if all the malignant features are present: infiltrative borders, high hypercellularity, stromal overgrowth, nuclear pleomorphism and more than ten mitotic figures/ten high power fields. If these changes are only localised to a small part of the tumour, the authors recommended calling the lesion borderline with possible metastatic potential [1]. On the other hand, the presence of malignant heterologous elements is enough by itself to label the lesion as malignant.

Benign phyllodes tumour differs from cellular fibroadenoma mainly by the presence of prominent leaf like structures, periductal stromal condensation, mild nuclear atypia and variability of the degree of stromal cellularity from one area to another. Pseudoangiomatous stromal hyperplasia and squamous metaplasia are more common in phyllodes tumours.

Benign multinucleated stromal giant cells can be present in phyllodes tumours and fibroadenomas. These are usually present in discrete groups and may show degenerative atypia with large hyperchromatic nuclei.

The distinction between benign phyllodes and cellular fibroadenoma in core biopsies can be difficult. A combination of stromal hypercellularity and heterogeneity, stromal sub-epithelial condensation, fragmentation of the cores, mitotic activity and nuclear pleomorphism are in favour of phyllodes, but unless these features are quite prominent, the lesion can be labelled as a cellular fibro-epithelial lesion and given a score of B3.

Distinguishing malignant phyllodes from metaplastic spindle cell carcinoma and breast sarcoma in core biopsies would rely on the presence of leaf like structures or benign glandular elements incorporated within the lesion. The presence of DCIS in the core would favour metaplastic carcinoma. Both phyllodes tumour and metaplastic carcinoma can show positive expression of p63 and cytokeratins, although these, when present, are more intense and diffuse in carcinoma. CD34 expression excludes metaplastic carcinoma [1].

Periductal stromal tumours: are considered variant of phyllodes tumours where there is isolated periductal stromal proliferation. These may be found near a proper phyllodes tumour or as separate nodules (Fig. 8.3).

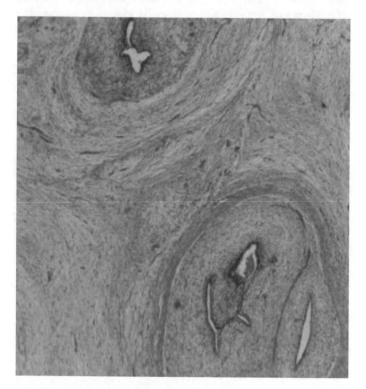

Fig. 8.3 Isolated peri-ductal stromal proliferation

Uncommon Breast Adenomas

Ductal adenoma: This is probably a variant of benign intraduct papilloma, where the epithelial proliferation is solid rather than papillary, and the lumen is totally obliterated [8, 9] (Fig. 8.4). Like benign intraduct papilloma the proliferating cells are a mixture of luminal and myoepithelial cells [10]. This can be confirmed by staining for CK5 which will show a mosaic pattern of staining.

Pleomorphic adenoma: These are uncommon well-circumscribed benign lesions present mostly in the peri-areolar region, suggesting an origin from large ducts [11]. They are usually single, but multiple lesions have been described. They can vary in size between 0.6 and 5.0 cm [11, 12]. Microscopically, they consist of a mixture of luminal and myoepithelial elements dispersed in a myxomatous or cartilagenous stroma (Fig. 8.5). A pseudo-capsules may be present around the lesion, but these may be penetrated by tumour tongues [11]. Immunohistochemically, focal positivity is

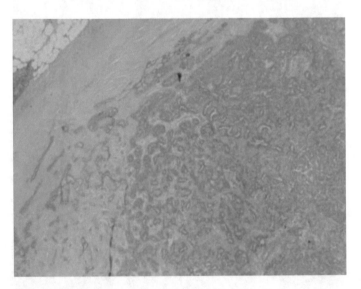

Fig. 8.4 Ductal adenoma

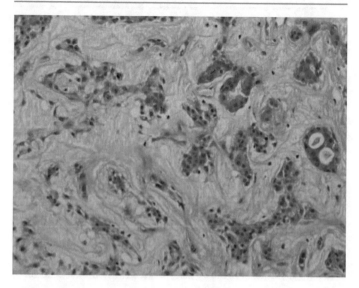

Fig. 8.5 Pleomorphic adenoma. A mixture of epithelial and myoepithelial cells in a myxomatous stroma

seen for ER and luminal and myoepithelial markers [11, 13]. Recurrence is unusual, but has been reported [14].

Nipple adenoma (Florid papillomatosis of the nipple) A benign lesion showing areas of usual type epithelial hyperplasia of variable degrees (Fig. 8.6). The lesion may be associated with erosion of the nipple, thus mimiking Paget's disease clinically [15]. The centre of the lesion may be sclerosed with entrapped small ducts, an appearance that can mimic tubular carcinoma. Benign cytokeratin 7 positive clear (Toker) cells [16] may be present in the epidermis overlying the lesion. These cells are HER2 negative (unlike Paget's cells which are HER2 positive) [17].

Syringomatous adenoma of the nipple: A rare benign but locally infiltrative lesion, similar to syringoma of the skin [18]. It has been described in women with ages varying between 28 and 74 years [18–20]. Microscopically, the lesion consists of tubular duct-like structures, cell nests and keratinizing cysts embedded in fibrous tissue [18, 19] (Fig. 8.7). The lesion does

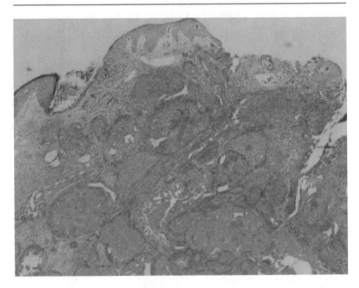

Fig. 8.6 Nipple adenoma ulcerating the overlying nipple skin

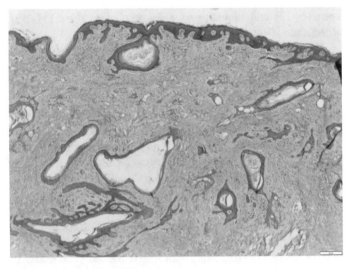

Fig. 8.7 Syringomatous adenoma of the nipple

not metastasise, but may recur [18]. Similar lesions have been described within the breast parenchyma away from the skin and the nipple [21].

Nodular hidradenoma: A small benign skin tumour of apocrine sweat gland origin which may rarely arise in the nipple/areola region or within the breast [22]. Microscopically, the lesion is well-circumscribed and consists of a cystic space containing proliferating epithelial and myoepithelial cells which may be arranged in papillary structures (hidradenoma papilliferum) or solid masses (nodular hidradenoma). Sometimes the lesion consists almost entirely of clear, presumably myoepithelial, cells.

Adenomyoepithelioma: An uncommon well defined benign solitary centrally located breast.

Lesion that radiologically resembles a fibroadenoma. The size varies between 1 and 7 cm. Microscopically, the lesion consists of scattered normal-looking breast ducts surrounded by marked proliferation of myoepithelial cells which compose at least 20% of the lesion's structure (Fig. 8.8). The myoepithelial cells could be spindle shaped, cuboidal with clear cytoplasm or rarely having an apocrine-like appearance with abundant eosinophilic cytoplasm. The dual epithelial myoepithelial nature of the lesion can be clearly visualised by immunohistochemistry using markers for myoepithelial cells, like p63 or CD10, which will show numerous positively stained myoepithelial cells surrounding unstained luminal epithelial cells lining the scattered ducts.

Malignant transformation can occur [7], hence it is advisable to give the lesion a B3 score when seen in a core biopsy. Malignant change is characterised by nuclear enlargement, hyperchromasia and abundant mitotic activity either in the myoepithelial or epithelial elements and could stay in situ or show evidence of invasion in the form of infiltrating cords or angulated cell clusters composed of cuboid or spindle cells [23, 24].

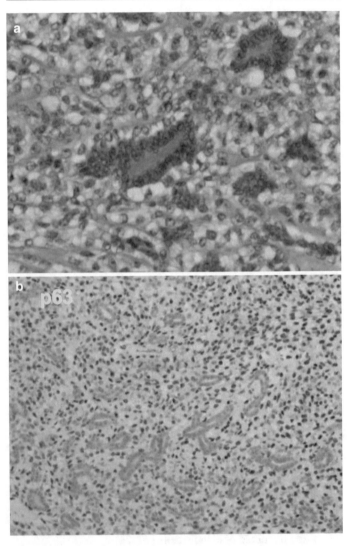

Fig. 8.8 Adenomyoepithelioma. (**a**) H&E showing well formed glands surrounded by myoepithelial cells with clear cytoplasm. (**b**) p63 showing positive nuclear staining of the myoepithelial cells

Pseudoangiomatous Stromal Hyperplasia

This is a benign proliferation of stromal fibrous tissue containing slit-like spaces that look like blood vessels but are devoid of endothelial cells as can be demonstrated by a negative staining for endothelial markers. It is common as an incidental microscopic finding and has been reported in 23% of 200 consecutive breast biopsies [25]. Occasionally, it may present as a mass lesion and can be multifocal [32]. In a series of 40 patients in whom the condition presented mainly as a palpable mass, the patients' ages varied between 14 and 67 years, with most of the patients being premenopausal or on hormone replacement therapy [26]. The cells stain for actin and desmin suggesting a myofibroblastic differentiation [26].

Diabetic Mastopathy

These are fibrotic breast lumps presenting in patients with long standing diabetes mellitus, more than 10 years, particularly the insulin-dependent variety. Patients usually have other diabetic complications or hypertension [27, 28]. The lesions vary in size between 2 and 6 cm, and are bilateral in 50% of cases. It can be seen in men as well as in women. Microscopically, there is dense fibrosis and heavy lobular and peri-vascular lymphocytic infiltration. 'Epithelioid' fibroblasts, sometimes multinucleated, may be present in the stroma (Fig. 8.9). The disease is self-limiting, but can recur. It has also been described in non-diabetic patients [29].

Silicon Mastitis and Breast Implant Associated Anaplastic Large Cell Lymphoma

Silicon can reach the breast tissue from an implant either through rupture or leakage. Microscopically, silicon is seen as unstained refractile irregular foreign bodies within cavities. These are usually associated with foamy histiocytes and foreign body giant cells.

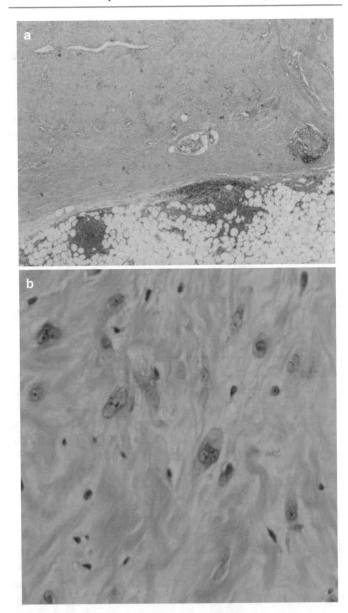

Fig. 8.9 Diabetic mastopathy (**a**) the lesion in this case was well circum-scribed and consisted of dense proliferation of fibroblasts/myofibroblasts and scattered lymphocytic aggregates. (**b**) High power view showing scattered atypical myofibroblasts

A heavy lymphocytic reaction is also commonly present. A similar reaction may be seen in draining axillary lymph nodes [30]. Older lesions will show extensive fibrosis which will form a 'capsule' around the implant [31]. The lining of the capsule may show partial or total mesothelial (synovial) [32] or epithelial (squamous) metaplasia [33]. Areas of ulceration with histiocytic reaction may occur in this lining, and rare cases of squamous cell carcinoma arising from the metaplastic epithelium have been described. Other local complications described with breast implants include lymphomas [34, 35], aggressive fibromatosis [36] and Kikuchi's histiocytic necrotizing lymphadenitis [37].

In particular, there has been widespread publicity about breast implant associated anaplastic large cell lymphoma, a sub-type of T-cell lymphoma that rarely occurs in the breast in the absence of implants. A review of 60 cases of this rare complication showed that 93% of patients with disease confined to the implant capsule achieved complete remission, compared with 72% of patients with a tumour mass [26]. It has been suggested that patients with disease limited to the capsule can be managed by limited capsulectomy and implant removal. Patients presenting with a mass have a more aggressive course that may be fatal justifying chemotherapy in addition to the removal of the implant [35].

Fat Necrosis

This is a relatively more common condition, usually occurring as a result of trauma which could be iatrogenic after surgical intervention. Grossly the breast tissue is indurated and show yellowish grey areas. Microscopically, there are empty, dissolved fat, spaces of variable sizes and sometimes cystic. These are surrounded by an inflammatory reaction composed of foamy histiocytes, lymphocytes and occasionally foreign body type giant cells. Evidence of recent or old haemorrhage with haemosiderin deposits, may be present. Older lesions also show fibrosis and sometimes calcification.

Fibromatosis

This is a non-encapsulated, infiltrative and well-differentiated fibroblastic lesion with an age incidence of 14–80 years. Microscopically, the lesion consists of bland spindle-shaped cells, arranged in long sweeping fascicles (Fig. 8.10). The degree of cellularity is variable. Mitotic figures are infrequent, but may be focally numerous . The lesion is usually stellate shaped with irregular extensions into adjacent tissue that may entrap breast ducts and acini. Immunohistochemically, the spindle cells stain positive for muscle specific and smooth muscle actin and show nuclear staining for beta catenin. Occasional cells may also be positive for desmin and S100. The lesion recurs in up to 27% of patients, but does not metastasis. The differential diagnosis includes nodular fasciitis, myofibroblastoma, fibrosarcoma and spindle cell (metaplastic) carcinoma [38–40].

Myofibroblastoma

An uncommon benign, non-recurring stromal tumour which can develop in men as well as women of all ages. The tumours can vary in size between 0.9 and 10 cm. Microscopically, the tumours are well-circumscribed and consist of spindle shaped cells arranged in short fascicles and clusters with bundles of collagen fibres dispersed in-between. No epithelial elements are present within the lesion. Mitotic figures are infrequent. Giant cells, fat cells, cartilage and myxoid areas may be present (Fig. 8.11).

Three variants have been described: collagenous, epithelioid and cellular. In the collagenous variant, collagen bundles predominate. In the epithelioid variant, 50% of the tumour consists of epithelioid cells arranged in alveolar patterns. The cellular variant consists of dense proliferation of spindle-shaped neoplastic myofibroblasts with cytological atypia; collagenous bundles may be absent in some parts of the lesion, and a peripheral infiltrative border may be present [41, 42].

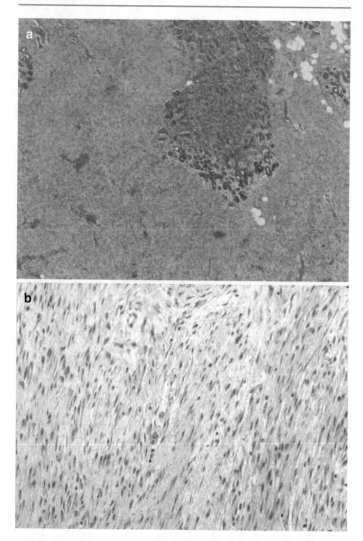

Fig. 8.10 Fibromatosis. (**a**) Proliferation of bundles of bland fibroblasts sweeping around, but not infiltrating, the breast glandular elements. (**b**) High power view of the fibroblastic bundles

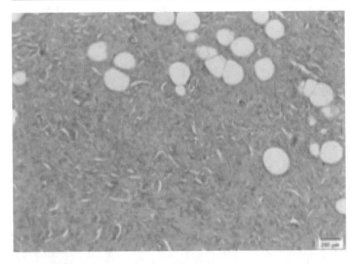

Fig. 8.11 Myofibroblastoma. Intermingles fibroblasts collagen fibres and in this case a few adipocytes

The tumours are negative for cytokeratin and the majority are positive for actin, desmin, vimentin, CD 34 and androgen receptors [40–43]. The differential diagnosis includes fibromatosis, nodular fasciitis, fibrosarcoma, spindle cell lipoma and spindle cell (metaplastic) carcinoma.

Nodular Fasciitis

These are well-circumscribed but not encapsulated lesions. Adjacent breast ducts and acini may be pushed aside by the lesion, but are not infiltrated . Lymphoid aggregates may be seen at the periphery. The degree of cellularity is variable, and focal collagenisation may occur in older lesions. Myxoid change is common and CD 68 positive osteoclast-like giant cells may be present. The central zone may be markedly hypocellular or even cystic. In early lesions, plump cells with prominent mitosis, but no artypia, are seen arranged in short fascicles and whorls in a loose myxoid matrix, resembling fibroblasts in tissue culture. The spindle cells, presumably myofibroblasts, are positive for muscle specific and smooth muscle actin and can be focally positive for desmin [43].

Ectopic Breast Tissue

Ectopic breast tissue, i.e. mammary glandular tissue present beyond the usual anatomic extent of the breast, is usually divided into two types: supernumerary breasts and aberrant breast tissue [44]:

- Supernumerary breasts refer to extra-mammary glandular breast tissue present along the milk line which extends from mid-axilla to the vulva. It is more commonly found in the axilla, and the overlying skin may show a nipple and areola.
- Aberrant breast tissue refers to mammary glandular tissue present beyond the usual anatomic extent of the breast or milk line. This usually becomes apparent only if it is involved in a pathological process.

Lesions, including carcinoma, arising from ectopic breast tissue within the axilla [45, 46], thoracic wall [47], and vulva [46, 48–51] have been described. There are also a few reports of lesions arising in aberrant breast tissue, outside the milk line, including the clavicular and anterior axillary regions, over the sternum, in the upper abdominal skin [44, 52]. We have also seen a case arising in the supraclavicular region.

To make a diagnosis of carcinoma arising in ectopic or aberrant breast tissue, in contrast to metastatic carcinoma, either normal or in situ malignant epithelial breast elements have to be present in coexistence with the lesion [44].

It has to be remembered that normal breast tissue may sometimes extend as a thin layer up to the clavicle [53] and beyond the infra-mammary fold. This explains why 'total' bilateral mastectomy in some patients, for example those with BRCA1 or 2 mutations, might not be enough to guarantee the removal of all breast tissue that may be susceptible to pathological changes [54], although admittedly the risk of carcinoma would be much reduced [55, 56].

References

1. Krings G, Bean GR, Chen Y-Y. Fibroepithelial lesions: the WHO spectrum. Semin Diagn Pathol. 2017;34(5):438–52. https://doi.org/10.1053/j.semdp.2017.05.006.
2. Silverman JS, Tamsen A. Mammary fibroadenoma and some phyllodes tumour stroma are composed of CD34+ fibroblasts and factor XIIIa+ dendrophages. Histopathology. 1996;29:411–9.
3. Kleer CG, Giordano TJ, Braun T, Oberman HA. Pathologic, immunohistochemical, and molecular features of benign and malignant phyllodes tumors of the breast. Mod Pathol. 2001;14:185–90.
4. Sawyer EJ, Poulsom R, Hunt FT, Jeffery R, Elia G, Ellis IO, Ellis P, Tomlinson IPM, Hanby AM. Malignant phyllodes tumours show stromal expression of c-myc and c-kit. J Athol. 2003;200:59–64.
5. Borhani-Khomani K, Moller Talman M-L, Kroman N, Tvedskov TF. Risk of local recurrence of benign and borderline phyllodes tumors: a Danish population-based retrospective study. Ann Surg Oncol. 2016;23:1543–8.
6. Cowan ML, Argani P, Cimino-Mathews A. Benign and low-grade fibroepithelial neoplasms of the breast have low recurrence rate after positive surgical margins. Mod Pathol. 2016;29:259–65.
7. Moo T-A, Alabdulkareem H, Tam A, Fontanet C, Lu Y, Landers A, et al. Association between recurrence and re-excision for close and positive margins versus observation in patients with benign phyllodes tumors. Ann Surg Oncol. 2017;24:3088–92.
8. Azzopardi JG, Salm R. Ductal adenoma of the breast: a lesion which can mimic carcinoma. J Pathol. 1984;144:15–23.
9. Lammie GA, Millis RR. Ductal adenoma of the breast—a review of fifteen cases. Hum Pathol. 1989;20:903–8.
10. Gusterson BA, Sloane JP, Midwood C, Gazet JC, Trott P, Taylor-Papadimitrious J, Bartek J. Ductal adenoma of the breast—a lesion exhibiting a myoepithelial/epithelial phenotype. Histopathology. 1987;11:103–10.
11. Diaz NM, McDivitt RW, Wick MR. Pleomorphic adenoma of the breast: a clinicopathologic and immunohistochemical study of 10 cases. Hum Pathol. 1991;22:1206–14.
12. Moran CA, Suster S, Carter D. Benign mixed tumours (pleomorphic adenomas) of the breast. Am J Surg Pathol. 1990;14:913–21.
13. Reid-Nicholson M, Bleiweiss I, Pace B, Azueta V, Jaffer S. Pleomorphic adenoma of the breast. A case report and distinction from mucinous carcinoma. Arch Pathol Lab Med. 2003;127:474–7.
14. Soreide JA, Anda O, Eriksen L, Holter J, Kjellevold KH. Pleomorphic adenoma of the human breast with local recurrence. Cancer. 1988;61:997–1001.
15. Diaz NM, Palmer JO, Wick MR. Erosive adenomatosis of the nipple: histology, immunohistology and differential diagnosis. Mod Pathol. 1992;5:179–83.

16. Toker C. Clear cells of the nipple epidermis. Cancer. 1970;25:601–10.
17. Zeng Z, Melamed J, Symmans P, Cangiarella JF, Shapiro RL, Peralta H, Symmans WF. Benign proliferative nipple duct lesions frequently contain CAM 5.2 and anti-cytokeratin 7 immunoreactive cells in the overlying epidermis. Am J Surg Pathol. 1999;23:1349–55.
18. Rosen PP. Syringomatous adenoma of the nipple. Am J Surg Pathol. 1983;7:739–45.
19. Ward BE, Cooper PH, Subramony C. Syringomatous tumor of the nipple. Am J Clin Pathol. 1989;92:692–6.
20. Slaughter MS, Pomerantz RA, Murad T, Hines JR. Infiltrating syringomatous adenoma of the nipple. Surgery. 1992;111:711–3.
21. Suster S, Moran CA, Hurt MA. Syringomatous squamous tumors of the breast. Cancer. 1991;67:2350–5.
22. Finck FM, Schwinn CP, Keasbey LE. Clear cell hidradenoma of the breast. Cancer. 1968;22:125–35.
23. Tavassoli FA. Myoepithelial lesions of the breast. Myoepitheliosis, adenomyoepithelioma, and myoepithelial carcinoma. Am J Surg Pathol. 1991;15:554–68.
24. Hayes MM. Adenomyoepithelioma of the breast: a review stressing its propensity for malignant transformation. J Clin Pathol. 2011;64:477–84.
25. Ibrahim RE, Sciotto CG, Weidner N. Pseudoangiomatous hyperplasia of mammary stroma. Some observations regarding its clinicopathologic spectrum. Cancer. 1989;63:1154–60.
26. Powell CM, Cranor ML, Rosen PP. Pseudoangiomatous stromal hyperplasia (PASH). A mammary stromal tumor with myofibroblastic differentiation. Am J Surg Pathol. 1995;19:270–7.
27. Tomaszewski JE, Brooks JSJ, Hicks D, Livolsi VA. Diabetic mastopathy: a distinctive clinicopathologic entity. Hum Pathol. 1992;23:780–6.
28. Seidman JD, Schnaper LA, Phillips LE. Mastopathy in insulin-requiring diabetes mellitus. Hum Pathol. 1994;25:817–24.
29. Ely KA, Tse G, Simpson JF, Clarfeld R, Page DL. Diabetic mastopathy. A clinicopathologic review. Am J Clin Pathol. 2000;113:541–5.
30. Truong LD, Cartwright J Jr, Goodman MD, Woznicki D. Silicone lymphadenopathy associated with augmentation mastopathy. Morphologic features of nine cases. Am J Surg Pathol. 1988;12:484–91.
31. Van Diest PJ, Beekman WH, Hage JJ. Pathology of silicone leakage from breast implants. J Clin Pathol. 1998;51:493–7.
32. Hameed MR, Erlandson R, Rosen PP. Capsular synovial-like hyperplasia around mammary implants similar to detritic synovitis. A morphologic and immunohistochemical study of 15 cases. Am J Surg Pathol. 1995;19:433–8.
33. Kitchen SB, Paletta CE, Shehadi SI, Bauer WC. Epithelialization of the lining of a breast implant capsule. Possible origin of squamous cell carcinoma associated with a breast implant capsule. Cancer. 1994;73:1449–52.

34. Cook PD, Osborne BM, Connor RL, Strauss JF. Follicular lymphoma adjacent to foreign body granulomatous inflammation and fibrosis surrounding silicone breast prosthesis. Am J Surg Pathol. 1995;19:712–7.
35. Niranda RN, Aladily TN, Prince M, et al. Breast implant-associated anaplastic large-cell lymphoma: long-term follow-up of 60 patients. J Clin Oncol. 2014;32(2):114–20.
36. Schiller VL, Arndt RD, Brenner RJ. Aggressive fibromatosis of the chest associated with a silicon breast implant. Chest. 1995;108:1466–8.
37. Sever CE, Leith CP, Appenzeller J, Foucar K. Kikuchi's histiocytic necrotizing lymphadenitis associated with ruptured silicone breast implant. Arch Pathol Lab Med. 1996;120:380–5.
38. Wargotz ES, Norris HJ, Austin RM, Enzinger FM. Fibromatosis of the breast. A clinical and pathological study of 28 cases. Am J Surg Pathol. 1987;11:38–45.
39. Rosen PP, Ernsberger D. Mammary fibromatosis. A benign spindle-cell tumor with significant risk for local recurrence. Cancer. 1989;63:1363–9.
40. McMenamin ME, DeSchryver K, Fletcher CDM. Fibrous lesions of the breast. Int J Surg Pathol. 2000;8:99–108.
41. Wargotz ES, Weiss SW, Norris HJ. Myofibroblastoma of the breast. Sixteen cases of a distinctive benign mesenchymal tumor. Am J Surg Pathol. 1987;11:493–502.
42. Rosen PP. Rosen's breast pathology. Philadelphia: Lippincott-Raven; 1997.
43. Morgan MB, Pitha J. Myofibroblastoma of the breast revisited: an etiologic association with androgen? Hum Pathol. 1998;29:347–51.
44. Rosen PP, Oberman HA. Tumours of the mammary gland. Washington, DC: Armed Forces Institute of Pathology; 1993. p. 20–1. & 270-272
45. Cogswell HD, Czerny EW. Carcinoma of aberrant breast of axilla. Am Surg. 1961;27:388–90.
46. O'Hara MF, Page DL. Adenomas of the breast and ectopic breast under lactational influences. Hum Pathol. 1985;16:707–12.
47. Livesey JR, Price BA. Metastatic accessory breast carcinoma in a thoracic subcutaneous nodule. J Roy Soc Med. 1990;83:799–800.
48. Guerry RL, Pratt-Thomas HR. Carcinoma of supernumerary breast of vulva with bilateral mammary cancer. Cancer. 1976;38:2570–4.
49. Cho D, Buscema J, Rosenshein NB, Woodruff JD. Primary breast cancer of the vulva. Obstet Gynecol. 1985;66:79S–81S.
50. Simon KE, Dutcher JP, Runowicz CD, Wiernik PH. Adenocarcinoma arising in vulvar breast tissue. Cancer. 1988;62:2234–8.
51. Rose PG, Roman LD, Reale FR, Tak WK, Hunter RE. Primary adenocarcinoma of the breast arising in the vulva. Obstet Gynecol. 1990;76:537–9.
52. Patrek J, Rosen PP, Robbins GF. Carcinoma of aberrant breast tissue. Clin Bull. 1980;10:13–5.
53. Holleb AI, Montgomery R, Farrow JH. The hazard of incomplete simple mastectomy. Surg Gynecol Obstet. 1965;121:819–22.

54. Eldar S, Meguid MM, Beatty JD. Cancer of the breast after prophylactic subcutaneous mastectomy. Am L Surg. 1984;148:692–3.
55. Meijers-Heijboer H, Van Geel B, Van Putten WLJ, Henzen-Logmans S, Seynaeve C, Menke-Pluymers MBE, Bartels CCM, Verhoog LC, Van Den Ouweland AMW, Niermeijer MF, Brekelmans CTM, Klijn JGM. Breast cancer after prophylactic bilateral mastectomy in women with BRCA1 or BRCA2 mutation. N Engl J Med. 2001;345:159–64.
56. Rebbeck TR, Friebel T, Lynch HT, Neuhausen SL, van't Veer L, Garber JE, Evans GR, Narod SA, Isaacs C, Matloff E, Daly MB, Olopade OI, Weber BL. Bilateral prophylactic mastectomy reduces breast cancer risk in BRCA1 and BRCA2 mutation carriers: the PROSE study group. J Clin Oncol. 2004;22:1055–62.

Women at Higher Risk of Developing Breast Cancer and the Concept of Risk-Based Breast Screening

9

Introduction

The aim of breast screening programmes is to catch carcinomas early enough to have a higher chance of conservative surgery and a higher chance of cure and survival. The 5-year survival for women with tumours less than 1 cm is 100% [1]. Mortality increases with increased tumour size and with the presence of more positive axillary lymph nodes. There is strong evidence that screening has reduced mortality from breast cancer. A large Danish study found an 11% reduction in mortality from breast cancer. However, a large number of deaths from breast cancer occurred in patients in whom the diagnosis of breast carcinoma was made when they were no longer eligible for screening. If this is taken into consideration the true reduction in mortality rate would be 20% [2].

However, screening has led to the problem of over diagnosis and over treatment as a result of subjecting large number of women to core and vacuum biopsies and sometimes to vacuum or surgical excision of benign or doubtful lesions. Hence a new concept of risk-based screening is developing as a result of an increased knowledge of breast cancer risk factors. This provides opportunities to shift from a one-size fits-all screening programme to a personalised approach, where screening and prevention are based on a woman's risk of developing breast cancer [3]. However, implementing such an approach presents challenges that have to be carefully considered. These include training for risk assessment and its communication to patients, the impact on work flow, psychological, ethical and legal and financial consequences [3].

Women at Higher Risk of Developing Breast Cancer

There are three main categories of women who would benefit from risk-based breast screening:

- Those with strong family history.
- Those in whom border-line breast disease; i.e. atypical hyperplasia and in situ lobular neoplasia have been diagnosed.
- Those with high mammographic density.

1. **Women at risk of developing breast cancer based on family history** [4]
   (a) The lifetime risk of developing breast cancer is around 12% for the general female British population.
   (b) Women who have relatives with a history of breast and/or ovarian cancer have a higher risk
   (c) The risk can be moderate or high
      - **Moderate risk (17–30% lifetime risk)** Patients have:
         – <u>One first degree relative</u> with breast cancer diagnosed before the age of <u>40</u> years.
         – <u>Two or three close relatives</u> with breast cancer at <u>any age</u> (at least one must be <u>a first</u> degree relative).
         – <u>Four close relatives</u> with breast cancer at <u>any age</u> (at least one must be a <u>second</u> degree relative)
      - **High risk (more than 30% lifetime risk)**

- Known breast cancer susceptibility gene mutation in the family (BRCA1, BRCA2, TP53)
- <u>One first degree relative</u> with breast cancer diagnosed at age less than <u>30</u> years
- <u>Two close relatives</u> with breast cancer diagnosed at an age less than <u>50</u> years (at least one must be a first degree relative)
- <u>Three close relatives</u> with breast cancer diagnosed at age less than <u>60</u> years (at least one must be a first degree relative)
- <u>Four close relatives</u> with breast cancer at <u>any</u> age (at least one must be a first degree relative)
- <u>One first degree relative with breast cancer at any age and any of the following</u>:
  - Bilateral breast cancer
  - Male breast cancer
  - Ovarian cancer
- Family history of Sarcoma diagnosed at age less than 40 years, brain, adrenocortical or any childhood cancer or multiple other tumour types at a young age.

2. **Women at risk of developing breast cancer based on history of: atypical hyperplasia and in situ lobular neoplasia** [5]:
   (a) These are present in around 5% of benign breast lesions
   (b) Life time risk is around 35%:
   (c) Risk increases with increase in number of foci
   (d) Risk the same whether or not there is a family history of breast cancer
   (e) Management: Tamoxifen for 5 years can be offered, but usually not taken.

3. **Women at risk of developing breast cancer based on increased mammographic density** [6]:
   (a) There is increasing evidence that mammographic density is a risk factor for the development of breast cancer.

(b) Comparing women at highest and lowest mammographic density yielded a fivefold higher risk of breast cancer for women at highest density.

(c) When adding microcalcifications and masses to the model, high-risk women had a nearly nine fold higher risk of breast cancer than those at lowest risk.

Management

Suggested mamnagement [4]:

1. **Follow up**
   (a) **Patients with <u>high risk</u>:**
      - **Annual mammography for >40 years**
      - **Annual MRI For <40 years**
   (b) **Patients with <u>moderate risk</u>:**
      - **Annual mammography or MRI until the age of 50**
      - **Then 3-yearly mammograms**
2. Chemoprevention for high risk women
   (a) **Tamoxifen for 5 years for pre-menopausal women (with no history of thrombo-embolic disease)**
      - **Tamoxifen for 5 years for post-menopausal women with no uterus (with no history of thrombo-embolic disease)**
      - **Raloxifen For 5 years for post menopausal women with a uterus**
      - **Effect of chemoprevention**
        - **50% reduction in breast cancer risk**
        - **Slight increase in endometrial cancer risk and thrombo-embolic disease**
        - **+ Other non-lethal side effects**
        - **Not all patients will tolerate tamoxifen.**
3. **Prophylactic mastectomy: for high risk patients with a very strong family history, Followed by immediate re-construction**

Uptake of Preventive Therapy in the UK

Uptake of tamoxifen is low in clinical practice. Only 1 in 7 women (14.7%) with increased risk of developing breast cancer who were offered the drug initiated the treatment. Women who had children were more likely to report taking the drug than those without children. Socio-demographic differences did not seem to have an effect on the rate of uptake [7].

References

1. Saadatmand S, Bretveld R, Sieslings S. Influence of tumour stage of breast cancer detection on survival in modern times: population based study in 173797 patients. BMJ. 2015;351:h4901. https://doi.org/10.11361/bmj.h4901.
2. Beay A-B, Andersen PK, Vejborg I, Lynge E. Limitations in the effect of screening on breast cancer mortality. J Clin Oncol. 2018;36:2988–94.
3. Rainey L, van der Waal D, Jervaeus A, Wengstrom Y, Gareth Evans D, Donnelly LS, Broeders MJM. Are we ready for the challenge of implementing risk-based breast cancer screening and primary prevention? Breast. 2018;39:24–32.
4. NICE clinical guidelines. CG 164. Familial breast cancer: classification, care and managing breast cancer and related risks in people with a family history of breast cancer. London: Nice; 2013.
5. Hartmann LC, Deglm AC, Santon WD, et al. Atypical hyperplasia of the breast-risk assessment and management options. New Engl J Med. 2015;372:78–89.
6. Eriksson M, Czene K, Pawitan Y. A clinical model for identifying the short-term risk of breast cancer. Breast Cancer Res. 2017;19(1):29. Published 2017 Mar 14. https://doi.org/10.1186/s13058-017-0820-y.
7. Hackett J, Thorneloe R, Side L, et al. Uptake of breast cancer preventive therapy in the UK: results from a multicentre prospective survey and qualitative interviews. Breast Cancer Res Treat. 2018;170:633–40.

Male Breast Biopsies

10

Introduction

Core and vacuum-assisted biopsies are usually carried out in male breasts as a result of breast enlargement or breast pain. They are dealt with in the same way as female breast biopsies and the spectrum of pathological changes, apart from gynaecomastia, are almost the same in male as well as in female breast. Thus, all types of in situ and invasive carcinomas, fibrocystic and columnar cell change, fibroadenomas, all types of benign and malignant papillary lesions, as well as soft tissue tumours particularly myofibroblastomas, have been described in the male breast and all show the same morphology and immunohistochemical profiles like those described in the female breast. Even gynaecomastia is not unique for male breast as 'gynacomastoid' hyperplasia is occasionally seen in the female breast. Hence we will concentrate here on the two main lesions affecting the male breast namely gynaecomastia and carcinoma, stressing the main features of the latter in the male breast.

Gynaecomastia

This is the commonest cause for enlargement of the male breast. It has to be distinguished from fatty breasts (lipomastia or pseudo-gynaecomastia). The latter has a soft consistency in contrast to the firm consistency of gynaecomastia induced by excess

© Springer Nature Switzerland AG 2020
S. Shousha, *Breast Pathology in Clinical Practice*, In Clinical
Practice, https://doi.org/10.1007/978-3-030-42386-5_10

fibrous tissue [1]. The condition results from an absolute or relative deficiency of androgen action or from excessive oestrogen action on breast tissue [1]. It is estimated that around 70% of pubertal boys develop a degree of breast enlargement which may persist in some into adulthood. This persistence accounts for around 25% of clinically presenting gynaecomastia. The cause of the disease in another 25% is unknown and in a further 25% the condition is drug induced. Other less common causes include testicular tumours (10%) and cirrhosis and malnutrition (8%) [2].

Microscopically two main types or phases of gynaecomastia are described: The florid type, reflecting recent onset and a fibrous type the quiescent inactive end stage of the disease (Fig. 10.1) [3]. A mixture of the two types may co-exist. Both types are characterised by ductal branching with epithelial proliferation which may be flat or micropapillary. The proliferating ducts are commonly lined by three layers of cells: an outer and inner CK5 positive ER negative, and a middle layer CK5 negative, ER positive (Fig. 10.2) [3]. In the early stage, the ducts are surrounded by a

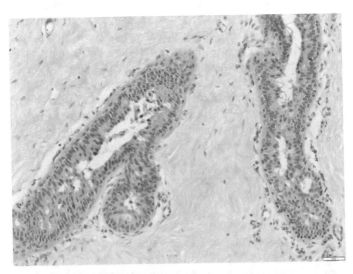

Fig. 10.1 Gynaecomastia, late fibrotic stage. Proliferative branching ducts surrounded by dense fibrous tissue (H&E)

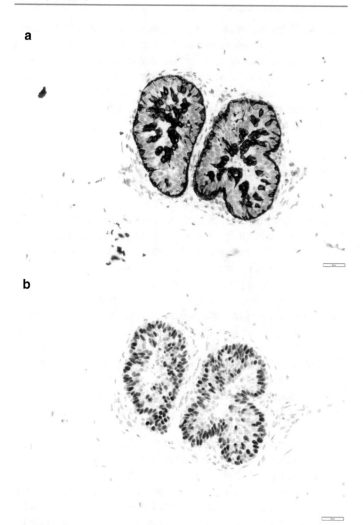

Fig. 10.2 Gynaecomastia, three layered epithelial hyperplasia. (**a**) Ducts stained for CK5 showing positive outer and inner layers and a negative middle layer. (**b**) ER staining show a strongly positive middle layer and negative outer and inner layers

highly cellular oedematous stroma that shows increased vascularity. Pseudo-angiomatous stromal hyperplasia may be present. The second later fibrous type, which is more commonly seen in practice, shows peri-ductal or confluent fibrosis with ductal proliferation and branching which are usually less than those seen in the early florid phase [3]. Gynaecomastia is not considered a precancerous condition.

Male Breast Carcinoma

Male breast cancer is a rare disease accounting for around 1% of all breast cancers. The epidemiology is similar to that of female breast cancer except that the majority of the inherited disease is due to BRAC2 mutations [4]. Other genetic factors include Klinefelter and Cowden syndromes, positive family history and Androgen receptor gene mutations [4].

Microscopically, the majority of male breast cancers, like female ones, are of the invasive ductal type. Invasive lobular carcinoma is less common than in female patients, but almost all other histological types are represented (Fig. 10.3). In a study of 1328 cases, 85% of tumours were invasive ductal, 1.4% invasive lobular, 5.5% mixed, 2.5% micropapillary, 1.4% mucinous, while the remaining cases included cribriform, adenoid cystic, invasive papillary, tubular, metaplastic, apocrine, secretory, sebaceous and clear cell carcinomas [5]. Around 50% were grade 2, 22% grade 1 and 27% grade 3. Around 85% were ER positive and 71% PR positive which is similar to female breast cancer, but HER2 was positive in only 2–10% of tumors, much less than that usually seen in female patients [5, 6]. One per cent were 'basal-like' and 0.2% were ER negative, PR positive [5]. Around 10% were under the age of 50 years, 62% between 50 and 75 and 27.5% above the age of 75 years. Thirty per cent of patients had positive axillary lymph nodes [5]. Around 45% of invasive ductal carcinomas had adjacent foci of DCIS, with both invasive and in situ elements having similar immunohistochemical and genomic features. The presence of associated DCIS appeared to be associated with a better outcome [5].

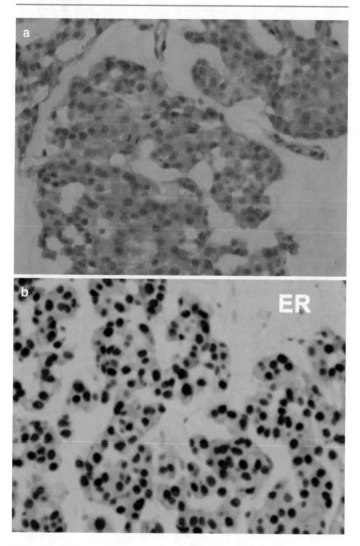

Fig. 10.3 (**a**) Invasive mucinous carcinoma developing in a 95-year old man and presenting as breast cyst. The tumour was ER strongly positive (**b**), p63 negative (thus excluding skin adnexal origin) and CK20 negative (excluding a metastasis from a colorectal carcinoma)

Of 347 male patients with breast cancer tested with oncotype DX, 21% had a high risk score compare with 14% of women tested during the same period [7]. Men with grade III and PR negative tumours are more likely to have a higher risk recurrence score and to receive chemotherapy.

References

1. Narula HS, Carlson HE. Gynaecomastia-pathophysiology, diagnosis and treatment. Nat Rev Endocrinol. 2014;10:684–98.
2. Braunstein GD. Gynaecomastia. N Engl J Med. 1993;328:490–5.
3. Kornegoor R, Verschuur-Maes AH, Buerger H, van Diest PJ. The 3-layerd ductal epithelium in gynaecomastia. Am J Surg Pathol. 2012;36:762–8.
4. Weiss JR, Moysich KB, Swede H, et al. Epidemiology of male breast cancer. Cancer Epidemiol Biomarkers Prev. 2005;14(1):20–6.
5. Doebar SC, Slaets L, Cardoso F, et al. Male breast cancer precursor lesions: analysis of the EORTC/10085/TBCRC/BIG/NABCG International Male Breast Cancer Program. Mod Pathol. 2017;30:509–18.
6. Humphries MP, Rajan SS, Honarpisheh H, et al. Characterisation of male breast cancer: a descriptive biomarker study from a large patient series. Sci Rep. 2017;7:45293. https://doi.org/10.1038/srep45293.
7. Altman AM, Kizy S, Yuan J, et al. Distribution of 21-gene recurrence scores in male breast cancer in the United States. Ann Surg Oncol. 2018;25:2296–302.

Index

© Springer Nature Switzerland AG 2020
S. Shousha, *Breast Pathology in Clinical Practice*, In Clinical
Practice, https://doi.org/10.1007/978-3-030-42386-5

Printed in the United States
By Bookmasters